"Dr. Leslyn Keith's new book, *The Lymphatic Code*, is brilliant! Though the lymphatic system is a major component of health and illness, it has been unfortunately neglected by the medical system. Dr. Keith's thorough yet simplified explanation of the lymphatic system, how it works, and what can help its optimum functioning lays the groundwork for ways to enhance one's health. Combining research with clinical experience, she lays out what you need to know to enhance treatment options for lymphatic disorders with nutritional solutions. Einstein said, "If you can't explain it simply, you don't understand it well enough." Dr. Keith understands the lymphatic system and related disorders more than well enough. *The Lymphatic Code* presents complex information clearly and simply for immediate application for those ready to transform their disease states to healthy living. It's groundbreaking in this field of study."

—CATHERINE SEO, PHD, FOUNDER & CEO, THE LIPEDEMA PROJECT,
LIPEDEMA SIMPLIFIED

"Being asked to write a review of this book is truly an honor. Not just because I support and believe in all the information in this book, but because I also believe in Leslyn. You will see as you read this book that she is trying to provide the patient the newest and most detailed information about the lymphatic system in a manner that is easy to understand and apply. She explains how a ketogenic lifestyle will truly improve a person's health. What I have learned and want you as a reader to understand is "the patient" to Leslyn is a friend, not just someone she treats. Leslyn truly cares and wants to see everyone living a healthy, happy life creating good memories. She understands how and where the traditional treatments for lymphedema fail and leave her patients hopelessly struggling, embarrassed, in pain and often owning the blame for this failure. She has witnessed how the ketogenic lifestyle turns everything around for her patients, giving them hope, building their confidence, and allowing them to become participants rather than spectators in the creation of memories with their friends and families. By allowing me to participate in life again, the ketogenic lifestyle has been of great benefit to me personally, and I encourage everyone to read this book and join me! Thank you Leslyn, for being there for me all these years and being my beacon of hope when I felt discouraged and alone in my fight. You are truly a wonderful person, and I am blessed to have you as a friend."

—KELLY BELL, LT

"The lymphatic system plays a vital, yet underappreciated, role in inflammation, immune function and general health. Dr. Keith has written an excellent book that explains normal and abnormal lymphatic function, with practical advice on what to do if you have lymphedema or lipedema. I highly recommend this book!"

— ERIC C. WESTMAN, MD MHS, DIRECTOR, DUKE KETO MEDICINE CLINIC, AUTHOR, END YOUR CARB CONFUSION

"As a person who is afflicted with lymphedema, I've learned how fickle, high maintenance and complicated it is – I live it every day. Dr. Leslyn Keith has graciously opened her mind, her studies, and her findings so we all don't have to keep fumbling around in the dark. Everyone who has it is different, their circumstances, their ages, but her comprehensive knowledge is a real shot in the arm for the entire lymphedema afflicted community."

—SEAN MULRONEY, THE OBESITY REVOLUTION PODCAST

"Leslyn never fails to astound me with her ability to thoughtfully research, analyze and deliver information in a manner that is engaging and accessible. She is always encouraging and inspiring, and I am a better clinician and my patients are more successful because of her. I have long admired Leslyn's passion to help her clients heal on the deepest level possible and she has outdone herself this time by creating comprehensive explanations of the lymph system, the mechanisms of lymphedema, and viable solutions for gaining control over lymphedema and lipedema."

—KAREN ASHFORTH, MS, OTR, CLT-LANA

"Dr. Leslyn Keith's first book, *The Ketogenic Diet for Lymphatic Disorders*, is such an important resource in my office, that I keep complimentary copies available for every client. My lymphedema clients who implement its principles noticeably improve in limb volume, tissue inflammation, and body composition. Dr. Keith's latest book, *The Lymphatic Code*, will certainly do for the general public, what her first book did for my lymphatically challenged clients. *The Lymphatic Code* maps out the benefits of the Ketogenic lifestyle including food choices, movement patterns, and relaxation techniques in an easy to read and implement format. I personally use these ketogenic principles in my own life to optimize health and healing. I can't wait to offer *The Lymphatic Code* to my clients so they may do the same."

—MICHELLE SANDERSON, CMT, CLT

"Although many diseases are associated with inflammation, research continues to show us that lipedema and lymphedema are particularly sensitive to inflammation and that diet can be a contributing factor. In *The Lymphatic Code*, Leslyn explores the complex subject of dietary science in relation to our lymphatic system and makes it easy to understand. She explains why maintaining optimal health requires a diet of complete proteins and fats, and she uses clear, easily understood concepts to dispel myths about the science of ketogenic diets in relation to not only our "Standard American Diet" but other popular diets as well. Leslyn's unique down-to-earth perspective on the multifactorial aspects of healthy habits for people with lymphatic impairments is also included in this book. She provides a comprehensive, common-sense perspective on positive physical and psychological habits that contribute to achieving and maintaining good health. This book, with its abundant resource lists, will help patients with lipedema and lymphedema gain confidence in using a ketogenic lifestyle as a tool to help control their weight, swelling and overall progression of their disease. *The Lymphatic Code* is a must read for those with lymphatic impairments!"

—LESLI BELL, DPT

"I will definitely recommend this book to my clients with lymphedema and other chronic illnesses. Leslyn has done an incredible job compiling the most recent evidence and research in a practical and applicable way. This book can be read as a whole and used as a reference guide for anyone that is interested in improved lymphatic and general health through lifestyle changes. Leslyn's methodical and scientific approach leaves no stone unturned. Her passion for new discoveries is evident. The lymphatic code is being cracked."

— ROBERT ERKSTAM, OTR, CLT, LANA

The Lymphatic Code

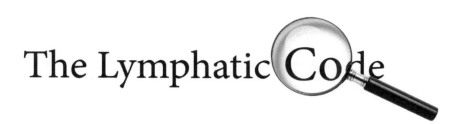

Using A Ketogenic Lifestyle To Enjoy A Robust
Lymphatic System That Promotes Overall
Health And Wellness

Leslyn Keith

Gutsy Badger Publishing
CHEYENNE, WY

The Lymphatic Code / Leslyn Keith
ISBN-13: 978-1-943721-19-1 (Paperback)
ISBN-13: 978-1-943721-20-7 (Electronic)

Dedication

RONALD JERRY DEMOSS
SEPTEMBER 19, 1958 – MARCH 7, 2021
TREASURED FRIEND
WHO INSPIRED ME TO UNDERTAKE
THIS JOURNEY IN NUTRITION AND LYMPHATICS

Acknowledgements

Ellen Davis, clinical nutritionist and editor extraordinaire

Catherine Seo, friend, colleague and galvanizing force

Robert Erkstam, lymphedema therapist and tremendous life coach

Kelly Bell, inspiring and determined lymphatic warrior

Bill Robinson, partner and phenomenal research assistant

Erin Keith, my favorite sister and fellow Carnivore

Table of Contents

Foreword

I met Dr. Leslyn Keith in San Luis Obispo, California, when I spoke at her low carb conference in 2014. The conference speakers included my colleagues and collaborators Dr. Eric Westman, Dr. Stephen Phinney, and Dr. Jeff Volek. This was at a time when conferences of this sort were not common and is testament to the fact that Leslyn is one of the pioneers in bringing this way of eating to the public. Her enthusiasm for using a low-carbohydrate, high fat ketogenic diet (LCHF/keto) as a therapeutic modality in her lymphedema clinic was intriguing at that time. At the conference she spoke to me of success among her clients who had adopted a LCHF/keto lifestyle. Many of these clients' conditions, including lymphedema and weight issues, improved. This was truly progressive at that time and unique in terms of a therapy for lymphedema.

A few years earlier, a diet study I had done was the subject of a documentary for CBC Television called My Big Fat Diet that Leslyn had seen on Youtube (where it might still be available). The study was done in the First Nations community of Alert Bay, on a small island off the coast of British Columbia. The premise was that a return to a traditional style, low-carb diet would be therapeutic for obesity and type 2 diabetes which are endemic in this population. The research subjects were mostly First Nations people but we allowed non-native residents to enlist as well. I found out later that one of these subjects had lymphedema which was markedly improved during the course of the study. He told me that his leg swelling had been so severe that he never wore shorts in public. After a few months on our low-carb study diet he no longer feared public exposure. So, of course, when Leslyn approached me with her plans for a conference I was happy to participate.

Over the ensuing years, Leslyn and her partner Bill began boating in south Puget Sound and, eventually made their way to the top of Vancouver Island where they could visit the study community in Alert Bay. Sometimes their itinerary involved stops in Horseshoe Bay, where my medical practice is located, with time for socializing. They were keenly interested in visiting the community in Alert Bay and to try the local traditional foods including oolichan grease, a unique marine fat that is a staple of the coastal First Nations diet.

As research on the benefits of LCHF/keto diet accumulates, we are beginning to understand its effect on a range of chronic metabolic and inflammatory conditions. Its benefits for overweight and type 2 diabetes are now widely recognized with authoritative guidelines starting to endorse this way of eating. In this context, the importance of nutrition's effect on the lymphatic system is only beginning to be recognized, largely through Leslyn's efforts. A few years ago, she ran a small pilot study among her lymphedema clients to explore how they might benefit from a LCHF/keto diet. The results were promising, suggesting that more research was needed to explore using LCHF/keto as an adjunct to existing lymphedema therapy modalities. Since then, Leslyn has been involved in other lymphatic studies using LCHF/keto diet methodology.

LCHF/keto is a safe and effective way of eating that has been proven to be beneficial for many conditions. It is also quite enjoyable. I have been eating this way since 2002 when I discovered I had type 2 diabetes. I am happy to report that my diabetes has been in remission over that time and that I maintain normal markers without the need for medications. It is somewhat puzzling, given the number of proven benefits that LCHF/keto can deliver, that it is not more widely adopted.

In *The Lymphatic Code*, Leslyn shows how this diet has profound effects on one of the most important systems in the body. Research on the lymphatic system and how it responds to dietary inputs has grown significantly in recent years. Leslyn presents this research and shows you how you can put it into practice to keep your lymphatic system healthy or to manage a lymphatic disorder.

I look forward to keeping up with Leslyn in the future as she continues to spread the message that using LCHF/keto is essential to keeping a well-functioning lymphatic system. And I look forward to their visits as they cruise the west coast in their twenty-eight foot Bayliner.

Jay Wortman, MD
July 2021
West Vancouver, BC

Preface

I am excited to bring to the lymphatic community another book about lymphatic health through dietary lifestyle change. My first book, *The Ketogenic Solution for Lymphatic Disorders: Lose Weight and Dramatically Reduce Lymphatic Swelling*, initially forged into nutrition to address weight control to allow better management of lymphatic disorders. It was directed primarily at lymphatic professionals to encourage them to incorporate nutrition in their practice. With a high percentage of patients with lymphedema and lipedema also suffering from obesity, I realized that weight management and nutrition couldn't be ignored if we wanted to help our patients achieve the best outcomes.

But two unexpected things happened. First, the book was more often read by individuals with a lymphatic disorder than by the practitioners who treat them. This meant that a book directed at the layperson was very much needed. The information must be clearly accessible and easily translated into action in order to help people with lymphatic disorders make successful lifestyle changes. Second, I have since learned that a ketogenic lifestyle means much more to lymphatic health than just weight loss. Many of my patients who adopted a ketogenic lifestyle were finding that their swelling and fibrosis were reduced, infections were less frequent or nonexistent, and they were able to wear compression garments less often even *when they didn't need to lose weight*.

I knew there was something else at work here. The great outcomes my patients were experiencing were more from changing to a healthy diet than they were about how many pounds they lost. Not that weight loss isn't important when needed, I've just come to understand that eating ketogenically is *more* important. Simply put: a ketogenic diet works for lymphatic disorders because **carbohydrates can be highly inflammatory, and fat fuels lymphatics**.

I also came to the realization that the state of our lymphatic system has a huge impact on our overall health. The medical community is only now realizing how important lymphatics are in health and disease. If you have a lymphatic disorder, consider taking this book to your clinician and asking if he or she would be receptive to adding proper human nutrition to your protocol. It is my sincere hope that what I have offered here will help you. Whatever you take from the advice in this book, I wish you all the best in your efforts to gain your best possible health.

The biggest take-away message from this book is that **healthy lymphatics equals a healthy life** and this is best achieved with a ketogenic lifestyle. I have learned so much in the process of writing this book. Come join me as we decipher the Lymphatic Code!

Introduction

"The game is afoot."
Sir Arthur Conan Doyle, Adventure of the Abbey Grange

The lymphatic system is made up of organized and complex pathways of vessels and specialized components, akin to the routes taken to discover all the clues in a Sherlock Holmes story. Sir Arthur Conan Doyle sent us down wide thoroughfares, narrow alleyways, gentrified streets and avenues, secret passages, dark hallways, and myriad other thruways in our efforts to decipher Sherlock's intricate cases. We, in our efforts to understand the lymphatic system and all its vessels and functions, must use the equivalent of Holmes's observation, deduction, scientific expertise, and reasoning skills to understand what the lymphatic system is and how we can help it accomplish its purposes. Come along with me as we gain insight into our abilities to keep our bodies healthy through proper functioning of the lymphatic system.

Although the lymph system is equally as extensive as the cardiovascular system, it is difficult to see, and has commonly been ignored or even disregarded, though it can be argued that it performs several times more functions than the cardiovascular system does. As we will see in Chapter 4, the ramifications of a poorly functioning lymphatic system are just as severe as an impaired cardiovascular system. Sadly, the lymphatic system is largely ignored in the medical training of most doctors. One survey found that a typical medical school curriculum includes less than thirty minutes of instruction on lymphatics.[1] Dr. Stanley Rockson, one of the authors of that study, noted that 14 years later the situation was no better. He was particularly distressed when he met with a patient who traveled many miles for answers regarding his hereditary lymphedema because his own medical providers from a large health care system did not know what to do for him. And because lymphatic disorders are so poorly recognized by the medical community, there are limitations on insurance coverage for treatments, which is even more discouraging.[2]

But changes are coming. General medical ignorance aside, in the past two decades there has been more scientific and medical research interest in the lymphatic system. It is now seen by those who are more informed as no less essential than the blood circulatory system[3] and is in actuality an elaborate immunovascular network. Professional associations and medical journals which had previously focused solely on veins are now interested in furthering research, supporting professional development and improving education about the lymphatic system in relation to the blood circulatory system. Founded in 1985, the North American Society of Phlebology officially changed its name to the American Vein & Lymphatic Society (AVLS) in 2019 to reflect the broadened scope and new focus on lymphatics. The National Institutes of Health (NIH) hosted its first symposium on the lymphatic system in 2015 and funding for research is now being encouraged. I was able to attend this inaugural symposium and presented my research on the use of a ketogenic diet (also referred to as keto or low carbohydrate in this book) for people with lymphedema and obesity. Interestingly, out of over forty poster presentations, mine was one of only two that used human subjects instead of animals in the presented research. We still have a long way to go!

In the Sherlock Holmes novels, evidence was hidden in plain sight, and you might say that the lymphatic system is hidden in plain sight as well. In *The Lymphatic Code*, I won't endeavor to keep clues hidden, since my purpose in this book is to explain what the lymphatic system does, and tell you what I have discovered that allows our lymphatics to operate at peak efficiency. This will, in turn, give you knowledge you need to keep your body in optimal condition.

I also intend to discuss lymphatic disorders such as cancer-related lymphedema, hereditary lymphedema, and lipedema so you might gain the ability to recognize some condition you or a loved one might have or develop. You will also learn to identify whether the condition has been caused by something that is within the power of the person to remedy, using the techniques I will present in this book. Unlike a mystery yarn, I intend to present you with facts that will help you get right to the information that will benefit you and your lymphatic system without sending you down useless distracting trails. So, let's go solve the case that Sir Arthur surprisingly never wrote, *The Case of the Historically Underappreciated Lymphatic System.*

Chapter 1

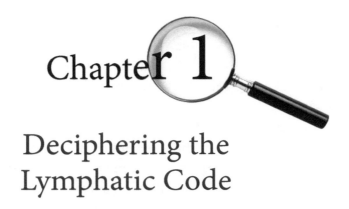

Deciphering the Lymphatic Code

"To begin at the beginning."
—*Sir Arthur Conan Doyle, A Study in Scarlet*

As soon as fluid from our tissues finds its way into a lymph capillary, it is called *lymph*. The origin of the word "lymph" comes from the ancient Roman deity *Lympha*, the goddess of water. She was considered highly consequential, as water was essential to agricultural success. Not only is this an apt characterization for this clear fluid, it also correctly indicates the significance of this system. The Latin word *lymphaticus* came to mean "connected to water."

The earliest known description of the lymphatic system was in the 5th century BC by Hippocrates and Aristotle.[4] Periods of discovery and illumination have been followed by longer periods of lamentable misinterpretations and relative obscurity. Although most medical schools have historically dismissed the lymphatic system as inconsequential, the importance of lymphatics in sickness and health has been gradually gaining ground in the current century. The slow progression of our knowledge is commonly ascribed to the transparent and delicate nature of the lymphatic system. Hippocrates, lauded as the father of medicine, identified the more easily visualized parts of the lymphatic system. These included *chyle*, the milky white lymphatic fluid found in abdominal lymphatics, as well as the lymph nodes located in the armpit, groin and neck.

Aristotle was able to describe *"fibers which take a position between blood vessels and nerves and which contain a colorless liquid."*[5] Gaspare Aselli, an Italian anatomist, "rediscovered" the lymphatic system in 1627 when he viewed "milky white" vessels in the gut of a dog that was dissected right after a meal.[3] It was not until the late 18th century that knowledge about the lymphatic system was expanded by Alexander Monro with his detailed anatomical description.[5]

Also pivotal in our understanding of the lymphatic system was the published theory by Ernest Starling in 1896 that described his view of how fluid in the tissues was returned to blood circulation.[6] Starling's Equilibrium supposed that most fluid was reabsorbed into the venous capillary, and the lymphatic system managed the overflow as a backup to the much more important cardiovascular system. This theory was undisputed for over 100 years until a revision was put forward by Levick and Michel in 2010.[7] Their research demonstrated the vital importance of the lymphatic system as the lymphatics are responsible for transporting almost *all fluid* from body tissues.

We see now that understanding the lymphatics and unraveling its code becomes another key to unlocking our understanding of human health. In order to understand the Lymphatic Code, we need to start with how the lymphatic system evolved, its embryonic development, and how it functions. Then we may begin to assemble the clues and build the evidence for what makes a healthy lymphatic system and why.

How We Lost Our Lymph Hearts

We vertebrates get our name from having a backbone, or a vertebral column. Thinking back to high school biology, we may recall that vertebrates are also distinguished from invertebrates by the fact that we have a skeleton on the inside of our body (rather than the skeletal armor found on the outside for insects), a nervous system and a developed brain. We now know that one other thing sets us apart: we have a lymphatic system.[8]

A rudimentary lymphatic system first appeared among vertebrates more than 450 million years ago in primitive jawless fish. The evolutionarily preserved lymphatic system in zebrafish, a present-day primitive vertebrate, has been invaluable in genetic research.[9] Essentially, it has been established that as vertebrates became larger in size over time, they needed not only a blood circulatory system to move nutrients around the larger body, they required a lymphatic system to remove and clean fluid and waste from tissues. Small invertebrates use diffusion to get nutrients to tissues and have no need for blood or lymphatic vessels. Larger invertebrates, like crabs, may have a primitive heart "which stir the fluid in open body compartments",[464] but still lack blood vessels or a developed lymphatic system.

Sometime in the transition from aquatic to terrestrial life, early vertebrates developed changes in their rudimentary lymphatic system. Little propulsion structures, called *lymph hearts*, were lost as land-dwelling mammals evolved. However, lymph hearts can still be observed today in amphibians, reptiles, and flightless birds, and they have improved our understanding of how our own system works. Evolution, it seems, went for a trade-off; we lost our lymph hearts and gained lymph nodes and a more highly developed immune system.[3]

The job of the lymph heart, to propel lymph against gravity, was retained in humans by our *lymphangions*, currently known as our "little hearts." The lymphangion is the segment between valves in a lymphatic vessel and is only present in

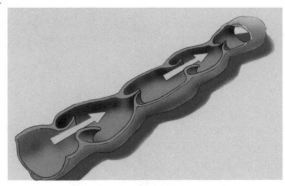

Figure 1. Fluid is propelled through the lymphatic vessels with rhythmic contractions of lymphangions.

the larger vessels, as we will see in Chapter 2. They have a combination of smooth and cardiac muscle that allows the vessel to rhythmically contract to push lymph along.[11] Both modern vertebrate lymph hearts and human lymphangions are responsive to increased pressure from lymph load (fluid in the tissues), intestinal peristalsis (contraction in the intestine during digestion), both passive and active movement of limbs, external pressure from compression or massage, and pulsation from nearby blood vessels.[12] Also influential on the pumping of lymphangions are changes in tissue pressure and increased lung volume, such as from deep diaphragmatic breathing.[13,14] Current practice uses this understanding of the evolutionary development of the lymphangion by incorporating abdominal pressure and deep breathing into the treatment of lymphatic disorders. The trained lymphedema therapist uses hand pressure to the abdomen coordinated with the patient's slow and full inhalation and exhalation to stimulate contraction of the lymphangion to increase the transport of lymph.

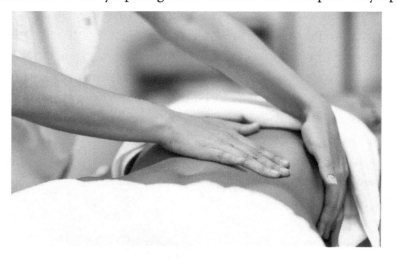

Figure 2. Hand pressure on the abdomen is coordinated with deep breathing to stimulate lymph flow.

Other evolutionarily preserved structures in the lymphatic system are the connection points between the lymphatic and blood circulatory systems.[15] Fluid is drained from the lymphatics into the right and left subclavian veins, just below the collarbone. Specialized valves are seen at these junction points that prevent blood from flowing backwards into the lymphatic system.[16] This is a common starting point in a variety of manual techniques used in treatment to facilitate the emptying of lymph into blood circulation. By starting at the end point, the lymphedema therapist can encourage emptying of fluid before stimulating more fluid to follow suit.

Effect of Deep Breathing

The responsiveness of lymphatic vessels to deep breathing throughout the body, not just in the trunk, was spectacularly demonstrated at a lymphedema conference several years ago. Dr. Eva Sevick-Muraca, a chemical engineer with training in biochemistry and biophysics, demonstrated the use of indocyanine green, a type of dye, for real time imaging of lymphatics. She injected the dye into the healthy arm of my friend and colleague Linda Roherty, a lymphedema therapist practicing in Tennessee. Observers were able to view the uptake of the dye into the lymphatics of Linda's arm and could easily discern lymphangion pumping and the gentle rate of progress of lymph toward her axillary nodes. Then Linda was instructed to take a few slow, deep breaths. Everyone in attendance was stunned to see the lymphatics in her arm begin to pump faster! *"I was amazed to see the lymphatic movement from deep breathing. I have a much greater respect for adding it to all HEPs [home exercise programs]."*

Consistently, throughout the evolutionary process, there has been a partnership between lymphatic and fat tissue. As mammals developed a more extensive lymphatic system, early lymph nodes and other lymphoid organs have always been embedded in fat tissue. In fact, researchers have observed an interesting phenomenon in lean mammals where prolonged fasting will deplete fat everywhere else on the body, but the fat surrounding lymph nodes is fully preserved.[17] Likewise, when fat surrounding lymph nodes is cut away, it will regenerate much more quickly than fat removed from areas remote from any lymph nodes.[18] The collaboration between fat (also called adipose or adipose tissue) and lymphatic tissue has beneficial implications for health that will be discussed further in Chapter 3 when we consider why a ketogenic diet is good for lymphatic health.

The lymphatic system in mammals, and especially in humans, has evolved to spectacular levels. There is more variety and specialization in our lymphatic system than in any other species.[19] Human lymphatic cells are able to differentiate depending on their location in the body and according to what their ultimate purpose will be. For instance, lymph cells near the intestine will specialize to become lacteals and will eventually carry essential fatty acids from the small intestine to blood circulation, while lymph vasculature in the skin will specialize to perform immune functions as a first line of defense against invading organisms.[20] Lymphatics are crucial for good health during the entire life cycle. For example, lung inflation and our first breath at birth wouldn't occur without the presence of specialized lymphatics in the lungs, and adult heart health, even after trauma such as a heart attack, is supported by the key role of cardiac lymphatics as well.[22]

Two Paths of Lymphatic System Development

Why is it important to understand how the lymphatics develop? If the mechanisms for *lymphangiogenesis* (lymph vessel generation) and embryonic development of the lymphatic system are understood, it can have amazing implications for both human health and disease. As will be discussed in Chapter 4, if we know how to stimulate or restrict the formation of new vessels, this may help us to treat many conditions such as lymphedema, Alzheimer's disease and cancer metastasis.

For example, when the lymphatic system has been impaired due to cancer treatment, lymphedema can develop. If new vessel development can be promoted and thus allow fluid to be transported out of a swollen area more efficiently, lymphedema may be more successfully treated or even prevented. Promoting lymphatic vessel formation can also help with removal of toxins and waste products in the brain to better manage Alzheimer's disease. Conversely, the restriction of vessel formation may reduce or even prevent cancer cells from metastasizing, or traveling to other parts of the body.

Groundbreaking work on the embryological development of the lymphatic system was performed by Florence Sabin while she was one of only fourteen female students at Johns Hopkins University School of Medicine in the years 1896-1900. Sabin, a pioneer for women in science, went on to become the first woman to become a full professor at a medical university. She furthered her research into the embryonic development of the lymphatic system while at Johns Hopkins and again later when working at the Rockefeller Institute for Medical Research. Her original theory, dubbed the Centrifugal Model, claimed that lymphatic vessels are formed from embryonic blood vessels. She and her colleagues suggested that lymph sacs sprout off of early veins centrally in the body and then grow to the periphery, eventually providing the developing fetus with a functioning lymphatic system.[23]

The Centripetal Model, introduced by Huntington and McClure in 1908, countered this view, advancing the idea that vessels germinate not from veins, but from other regional tissues. George S. Huntington was a medical doctor and the first full-time anatomy professor at a medical university. He transformed how anatomy was taught, by making the subject lab-based instead of being situated in the traditional lecture hall. Huntington, fascinated by the comparison of anatomical features between different species, shared his interest in comparative anatomy, embryology, and morphology with Charles F. W. McClure, a renowned researcher and professor at Princeton University.[24] Their Centripetal model argued that lymph vessels arose out of mesenchymal cells, or primitive cells that could develop into connective tissue, blood vessels, or lymphatic vessels, depending on need. Huntington and

McClure contended that lymphatics did not originate centrally and spread out, as Sabin suggested, but rather emerged from local tissues throughout the body.

The controversy between these two opposing views of how the lymphatic system develops has continued into this century.[25] Both theories' proponents were criticized for using faulty methods, however recent advances in research methodology and imaging have enabled us to learn that the lymphatic system actually uses both methods for its early development.[15] It has now been theorized that the method of lymphatic development is organ specific. In other words, the type of embryonic lymphatic generation, whether centrifugal or centripetal, depends on which tissue the budding lymphatics will be used for, such as the intestine, the skin, or the heart.[20] Lymphatic vessels attain special characteristics that are needed in the environment in which they are found. As our understanding of the unique organ-specific characteristics of lymphatics improves, this may help us treat many common diseases in which we now understand that the lymphatic system plays a major role. I will discuss these new discoveries further in Chapter 4.

What instigates the budding of lymphatic vessels and structures in the first place? Researchers have isolated various genes that are involved in the formation of the lymphatic system such as Prox1, and various vascular endothelial growth factors (VEGF). Increased expression of key genes or lymphatic biomarkers is correlated with periods of differentiation and lymphatic growth.[26] This is a process that begins in the fifth week of gestation with rapid lymphatic growth continuing through puberty. Further growth and development of the lymphatic system can occur throughout the lifespan, but this process has been studied very little except in the context of lymphangiogenesis associated with cancer.[27]

Can our diet also stimulate lymphatic growth and development? Humans have evolved to successfully and efficiently use several alternative energy sources. Among these are glucose, fatty acids and ketones. Our lymphatic system is similar in its energy usage, and may even preferentially use fatty acids and ketones.[28] Recent animal research has shown that fatty acid metabolism and ketone supplementation stimulates lymph vessel growth.[29,28] A human case study report demonstrated that, if no other source of fatty acid were available, the lymphatic system will absorb medium chain triglycerides which are never found in lymph under normal circumstances.[30] The only case report of an infant spontaneously resolving congenital lymphedema in his leg in his first year of life may have occurred due to lymph vessel formation promoted by fatty acids and ketones introduced through breast feeding, although no information regarding his or his mother's diet was available.[31] Further knowledge about what stimulates lymphatic vessel growth could have a profound impact on the treatment of lymphatic disorders such as lymphedema and lipedema.

As we continue on our journey to decipher the *Lymphatic Code*, lymphatic anatomy and function must be explored. These topics will be discussed in the next chapter.

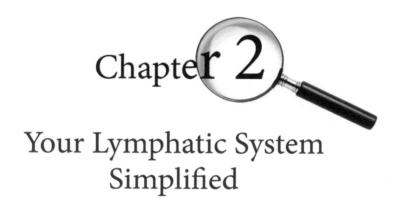

Chapter 2

Your Lymphatic System Simplified

"Pshaw, my dear boy! [I]t was simplicity itself."
—*Sir Arthur Conan Doyle, The Sign of the Four*

To continue on our journey of deciphering the Lymphatic Code, we will need to better understand the fascinating anatomy of the lymphatic system. As we uncover the mysteries of this system, it is almost like discovering how a spectacular trick is performed by a master magician. Once we have seen how the feat is done, everything falls into place and seems so obvious. Why have we not seen and understood this before? But no matter. The somewhat arduous journey to comprehend both the beguiling complexity and the artful simplicity of the lymphatics makes it that much more interesting.

Imaging the Lymphatics

Improvements in lymphatic vessel and structure imaging have greatly increased our knowledge of lymphatic anatomy and function, and this helps guide intervention and treatment. One of the best ways to understand the lymphatic system is to visualize it in a living creature. These living visualization techniques are also used in research to understand lymphatic system development and function and to better understand clinical lymphatic abnormalities and cancer metastasis. For certain lymphatic impairments, proper imaging is an absolute necessity to guide proper treatments and, in some cases, even possible resolution of the dysfunction.[32] Described here are the most commonly used techniques for imaging the lymphatics.

The standard imaging employed for decades was lymphography, or *lymphangiography*, until adverse complications from this technique were observed in patients, and alternative techniques with better image resolution were found. Developed by Kinmonth in 1952, lymphangiography is highly invasive, requiring multiple injections, and is time consuming.[33] This technique is still noted to be superior for finding malignancies. It is often used in conjunction with computed tomography (CT) scans by some radiologists when cancer is a concern.[34] Magnetic resonance lymphangiography (MRL) also combines two technologies, and it has been useful as well as less invasive than traditional lymphangiography for diagnosing lymphatic abnormalities. MRL has the added benefit of not requiring the use of ionizing radiation.[35]

A much more common lymphatic imaging technique is the use of lymphoscintigraphy, also called *lymphangioscintigraphy*. A radioactive tracer is injected in the skin, usually on the foot or hand. Images are taken over a period of several hours to give a general impression of the state of lymphatic functioning. Unfortunately, due to very poor resolution, this technique can't show the location and appearance of nodes and vessels.[33] For this reason, lymphangioscintigraphy may be combined with other imaging techniques such as CT scan, positron emission tomography (PET) scan, or magnetic resonance imaging (MRI).

Newer imaging techniques utilizing near-infrared (NIR) fluorescence, such as *indocyanine green (ICG)*, allow a real time visualization of the contraction of lymph vessels and location of lymph nodes. ICG is less invasive than lymphoscintigraphy and does not require exposure to radiation. This technique is being developed for use in clinics to help guide treatment of lymphatic disorders. ICG is somewhat limited, though, by the visibility depth of just two centimeters.[36] ICG is somewhat limited, though, by the visibility depth of just two centimeters and is ineffective for visualizing the deeper central lymphatics of the trunk.

Another lymphatics imaging technique is *contrast-enhanced ultrasound (CEUS)* which uses a contrast agent along with sound waves to visualize lymph nodes and vessels. This imaging method is particularly useful in diagnosing lymphatic dysfunction in the trunk.[32] New options on the horizon for lymphatic imaging include *optical frequency domain imaging (OFDI) and optical coherence tomography (OCT).*[33]

Despite the limitations of current imaging techniques, visualization of the lymphatics has created the basis of most of what we know about this intriguing body system. It is exciting to contemplate that as new advances in lymphatic imaging are made, more accurate identification of dysfunction will inevitably result in more effective treatments for those issues. Ultimately, this will vastly improve the health outcomes for many people with a lymphatic disorder.

Sleuthing Lymphatic Anatomy

The human lymphatic system is an extensive network that reaches nearly every part of the body. If we were to strip away the rest of the body's tissues leaving only the lymphatic vessels and organs, we would see a completely recognizable human form. Until recently, it was supposed that certain parts of the body were not served by lymphatics, such as the brain, spinal cord, eye, bone marrow, cartilage, and inner ear. With the discovery of *glymphatics*, we now know the central nervous system (brain and spinal cord) are served by specialized lymphatics[37] as is the inner ear.[38] While immature lymphatic structures in the bone and bone marrow are normal, fully developed structures and complete infiltration of lymphatics into this area is not. Fully mature lymphatics in these regions is actually a sign of pathology.[39,40] Currently, cartilage seems to be the last holdout without any lymphatics, relying completely on diffusion for nutrient supply and waste removal.[41]

In order to best understand the anatomy of the lymphatic system, let's follow a drop of fluid as it navigates its way through this incredible system and finally re-enters the blood circulatory system. It is always beneficial to get an overview of where we are going by looking at a roadmap first. On this trip, our droplet is bringing nutrients from the blood plasma into the surrounding cells and tissues. Although the diagram below doesn't show us all of the smallest lymphatic channels, the major thoroughfares and highways that are depicted give a nice outline of where our drop of fluid can travel and what its ultimate

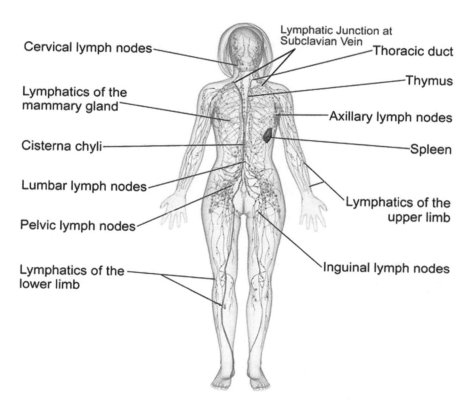

Figure 3. Overview of the lymphatic system. (front view). Red line is the route of our droplet of water.

destination might be. Our droplet of water in this example will travel from tissue in the foot, through the lymphatic system, and then finally back into the blood via the junction of the *thoracic duct* to a major vein near the left collarbone.

Arterial Blood Capillary: Our Droplet Moves from the Bloodstream to Nourish Tissues.

Our trek begins as our droplet of water squeezes through a tiny opening in a tiny blood vessel called an *arterial capillary* and flows into the space between cells in the surrounding tissues (the *interstitial space*). Its job at this point is to provide nourishment to the local cells. The amount of leakiness of a blood capillary depends on its location in the body. The most common blood capillary is *continuous* and only allows water or ions (very small particles) to exit. *Fenestrated* capillaries have slightly larger openings and *sinusoid* capillaries are the leakiest.

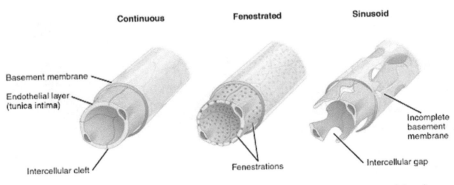

Figure 4. Three types of blood capillaries. The most commonly occurring of the three are continuous capillaries.

The inside of all blood vessels, including capillaries, are lined with a delicate gel-like barrier layer called a *glycocalyx*. The gel covers and protects a carpet of tiny hair-like extensions attached to the vessel lining. The glycocalyx functions as a gatekeeper, deciding which particles and how many are allowed to exit the vessel.[42] However, the glycocalyx is easily damaged by hyperglycemia, or high levels of blood glucose, which is amply supplied by a diet high in carbohydrates. This damage results in excessive leakage of fluid into bodily tissues.[43] A healthy glycocalyx is especially important for people with lymphatic disorders because too much fluid leaking out of blood capillaries can cause or worsen swelling.

Once oxygen and other nutrients have been delivered to the local cells, our water droplet needs to enter a lymph capillary to be evacuated. We now know that, except for limited special situations, almost 100 percent of the fluid evacuated from the tissues is transported by the lymphatic system to eventually join the bloodstream, and virtually nothing is reabsorbed into the venous capillaries.[7] It is interesting to note that the very act of gaining entrance to the lymphatic system constitutes the formation of lymph. Until fluid and particles enter the lymphatic system, it is not called lymph, and instead is termed *interstitial fluid*. Lymph may contain water, glucose, salt, fat, protein, dead or damaged cells, white blood cells, and other debris depending upon where it originates. The composition of lymph will be very different, for instance, if it comes from muscle, subcutaneous fat, or the intestines.

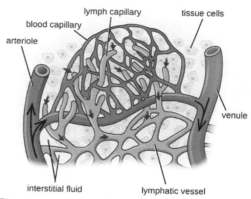

Figure 5. Microcirculation with blood and lymph capillaries for delivery and evacuation of fluid and particles from tissues.

Lymph Capillaries: Our Droplet Enters the Lymphatic System.

While the arterial capillary is barely big enough at 5-10 microns for red blood cells to move along in a single file, the lymphatic capillary is much larger at 20-30 microns. This accommodates fluid as well as larger particles and debris. The lymph capillaries are the most delicate of all lymphatic vessels. Their walls are made up of single overlapping cells which operate like flaps that open to allow fluid to enter into the capillary but not exit. These cells are tethered to surrounding tissue by specialized *anchoring filaments*. Anchoring filaments prevent lymphatic capillaries from collapsing and also act to open the cellular flaps to allow fluid entrance.[44]

Lymphatic Capillary

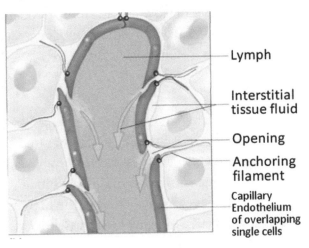

Figure 6. Lymphatic capillary showing anchoring filaments and path of interstitial fluid.

What encourages our water droplet to enter the lymph capillary? One theory is that increased pressure in the tissues *pushes* fluid into the lower pressure lymph capillary. Increased tissue pressures can arise from muscle contraction, pulsation of nearby blood vessels, compression, massage and fluid accumulation in the tissue itself. An opposing theory is that the relaxation phase after contraction of lymphangions in the larger lymphatic vessels creates a negative pressure and sucks or *pulls* the fluid into the lymph capillary.[45] In practice, intervention and management of a lymphatic disorder will take advantage of both of these theories with the use of manual lymph drainage, compression therapy, exercise and deep breathing.

Pre-Collectors.

Our water droplet next travels into a lymphatic pre-collector. These vessels are a hybrid between a lymph capillary and the larger lymphatic collectors, intermittently containing flaps seen in the capillary that allow fluid to enter the vessel, but also having sporadic appearances of the muscle and one-way valves of the lymph collectors. Thus, the pre-collector can both absorb and propel fluid.[46] As our drop of water nears the next larger lymphatic vessel, the walls become more continuous and absorb less fluid. The presence of valves occurs more frequently and they display a more concerted effort to propel fluid with contractions of the smooth and cardiac muscle in the walls of the vessel.

Lymph Collectors.

Our journey continues with our water droplet flowing into a lymphatic collector and from there making a trek from the foot to the back of the knee through this vessel. A collecting vessel is larger than either a lymph capillary or pre-collector, measuring 1-2 millimeters in diameter. There are other important differences as well. We see the first appearance of a lymphatic glycocalyx, similar to the blood vessel glycocalyx, in the collecting vessels. One of the important functions of the lymphatic glycocalyx is to make a super slippery surface that keeps immune cells rolling along by preventing them from sticking to the vessel wall. The glycocalyx functions similarly in a lymph vessel as it does in a blood vessel: namely as a gatekeeper, as it carefully regulates interaction between the lymph vessel and surrounding tissues.[47]

As our droplet traverses the lymphatic collecting vessel, we also note that the appearance of one-way valves is more common, and the vessel wall is consistently sturdy with smooth and cardiac muscle. Our water droplet is propelled through the lymph collector by lymphangion contraction, as discussed in Chapter 1. With each contraction, the lymphangion shrinks and pushes its contents into the next lymphangion. During relaxation, a lymphangion can distend tremendously, doubling or even tripling size, allowing the influx of more lymph.[46] Contraction rate, dependent upon the fluid load in the tissues, can range from six to ten times per minute to as much as ten times that rate when needed.[48] Lymphangion contractions are coordinated, purposeful, and highly effective in propelling the droplet against gravity up the calf, stopping momentarily at the lymph nodes behind the knee, then continuing up the thigh through another lymphatic collecting vessel, and finally to a lymph node depot at the groin.

Lymph Nodes.

There are approximately 600 lymph nodes in the human body, most of which are in the abdomen. Small groups of nodes can be found in the subcutaneous tissue in various regions in the body such as the underarm, groin, crook of the elbow, and behind the knee. We are most familiar with those at the sides of the neck, especially when they are enlarged when we are ill. Most lymph nodes lie in a bed of fat that is believed to function as a convenient source of fuel.[49] Lymph nodes can vary in size from 2 millimeters (a very small ball bearing) to 2 centimeters (a blueberry). As our droplet of water travels up the leg, it will pass through the nodes behind the knee (*popliteal nodes*) and those at the groin (*inguinal nodes*).

Lymph nodes have two primary functions: assist the immune system and filter lymph. As our water droplet proceeds through the popliteal and inguinal lymph nodes, it is screened for bacteria, parasites, viruses and other noxious particles. Lymph nodes store white blood cells, or *lymphocytes* (immune cells that are trained to recognize certain foreign matter and build an immune response). Lymph nodes also filter lymph to rid it of waste products, dead cells, and even cancer cells, using *macrophages* to engulf and eliminate any invaders.

Lymphatic Trunks and the Thoracic Duct.

The largest lymphatic vessels in the body are called the lymphatic trunks. As our water droplet passes through the inguinal nodes at the groin, it will enter the *lumbar trunk*, continuing to be propelled upward by lymphangion contraction. Further filtration of the lymph fluid carried in the trunks will occur in the deep pelvic nodes as our drop of water travels onward.

The right and left lumbar trunks exit the right and left legs respectively and join at the *cisterna chyli*, an enlarged sac that constitutes the beginning of the *thoracic duct*. Lymphatic vessels draining organs, most notably the liver, heart, lungs and intestine, also feed into the cisterna chyli. The thoracic duct can be up to forty centimeters long (about 17½") starting just above the level of the belly button with the cisterna chyli, penetrating through the diaphragm, and extending to the base of the neck near the left collarbone. The thoracic duct is the largest lymphatic trunk with a diameter of 2-5 millimeters. This size is required because three quarters of the lymph in our body is transported by the thoracic duct. All fluid from the lower body to the waist, the left side of the trunk, left arm, and left side of the head and neck is drained into the thoracic duct. The thoracic duct must also accommodate any chyle, the milky white fluid mentioned in Chapter 1,

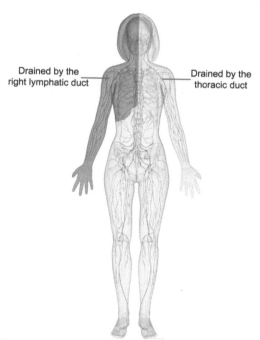

Drained by the right lymphatic duct

Drained by the thoracic duct

Figure 7. Seventy-five percent of the body drains into the thoracic duct, while the remaining twenty-five percent enters the right lymphatic duct.

that is picked up from the intestinal lacteals. The *right lymphatic duct* manages the fluid from the remaining areas including the right side of the trunk, right arm, and right side of the head and neck (see Figure 7).

The uppermost portion of the thoracic duct connects with the subclavian vein to form the junction with the blood circulatory system. This portion of the thoracic duct is often slightly enlarged and contains secondary valves that prevent venous blood from entering the lymphatic system. Higher pressure in the thoracic duct compared to that of the subclavian vein encourages lymph to flow in the correct direction.

The discussion in Chapter 4 covers cardiovascular conditions, including venous hypertension, which can inhibit the emptying of lymph into the venous system and create swelling. These conditions can be a major cause of breathing difficulties. The thoracic duct can be vulnerable to injury from surgery and other medical procedures to the neck and trunk, most particularly those performed on the esophagus. Complications from thoracic duct injury can include swelling, pain, difficulty breathing, gastrointestinal distress, and nutritional deficiencies.[50] This was the case for Kelly Bell when he went in for a simple procedure to treat a hiatal hernia that involved injecting a polymer into his esophagus. Disastrously, polymer also went into his thoracic duct:

> *"I had a simple medical procedure for a hiatal hernia and acid reflux ... a liquid polymer bulking agent that was injected endoscopically at the lower esophageal sphincter to close off the hernia... I received a CT Scan where I was told the polymer was everywhere. It was in my liver, spleen, right lung, a large chunk in the center of my chest, around my intestines, and in the lymph nodes at the top of my stomach... I required surgery to remove the middle lobe of my right lung... My pulmonary issues progressed to the point where I was put on oxygen and I developed stage 3 congestive heart failure. It became extremely difficult to walk even a mile, let alone the athletic events I used to compete in, because of the lack of oxygen [and] difficulty in breathing." —Kelly B.*

Lymphoid Organs.

There are several specialized organs that are considered part of the lymphatic system, but their association is not obvious. These lymphoid organs include the thymus gland, spleen, tonsils, *Peyer's patches*, and bone marrow. These organs primarily assist the lymphatic system with immune function. The thymus gland lies in the upper chest just behind the sternum and is responsible for developing *T-lymphocytes* to fight specific pathogens. The spleen, located in the upper left abdomen, is filled with lymphocytes and macrophages which can be quickly deployed to fight an infection or other invading bodies. Tonsils also mount an immediate defense and are well-placed in the throat to attack any invaders that enter the body through the mouth. Peyer's patches are lymph node-like organs in the lining of the small intestine that test food for toxins and initiate an immune response if needed. Lastly, bone marrow is integral to immune demand with its ability to develop both general and highly specific immune cells.

We followed the journey of a droplet of water as it traveled through the lymphatic system from the foot to the thoracic duct and into the blood circulation. Lymph fluid, in the same manner, would be transported no matter where it originates in the body. Fluid and particles are transported through gradually larger and larger vessels and filtered in the lymph nodes until a much improved product is deposited into the blood. Now that we have a better understanding of lymphatic anatomy, let's continue unravelling the Lymphatic Code by learning about the functions of the lymphatic system.

Investigating Lymphatic System Function

The lymphatic system has several important tasks that have typically not always been judged significant... until a malfunction occurs. While the work of the lymphatic system is crucial to human health and optimal functioning, it performs its job in such a quiet and efficient manner that it has consequently gone almost unnoticed. Here, we continue our work of interpreting the Lymphatic Code by discussing and exploring those vital functions.

Fluid Balance and Waste Removal.

As discussed previously, recent research supports the view that almost all fluid in the tissues can be delivered back into blood circulation only by the lymphatic system.[7] This concept is still poorly accepted by the medical community, however. It is not unusual to read an article stating that one function of the lymphatics is to remove 'excessive' fluid or even simply 'residual' fluid. The lymphatic system is still considered by many to be merely a back-up to the more important cardiovascular system.

The truth is much more interesting. Capillaries, which form a major portion of the cardiovascular system are riddled with fenestrations, or holes, through which fluid and very small particles can pass. Triglycerides, carried by lipoproteins such as chylomicrons, and other nutrients pass freely out of the small arteries into the interstitial spaces to be taken up as needed by the cells of the body. What cannot pass through these tiny fenestrations are corpuscles (blood cells), which make up about half of the volume of blood. Corpuscles are many thousands of times larger than the other nutrients and particles floating in the blood. The clear fluid in which corpuscles travel through the arteries or veins is known as blood plasma. Once this fluid is taken up by the lymphatic system, however, it is known as lymph.

During every minute of every hour, approximately one percent of the blood plasma leaks through these fenestrations into the interstitial space. So that means that every hour and a half or so, the equivalent of one-hundred percent of the fluid in the blood leaves the cardiovascular system and flows into the lymph system. The lymphatic system eventually returns that fluid to the cardiac system through the thoracic duct. This mechanism gives us a whole new perspective on the importance of the lymphatic system.

Maintaining a fluid balance in the body is required for life. Thankfully, the total capacity of the lymphatic system to meet the needs of fluid transport can be as much as twenty times what is needed under normal conditions.[51] In a healthy person, increased fluid volume in tissues can occur as much as several times per day. This is easily accommodated by the lymphatics – if not immediately, then usually at least within several hours, by increasing the contraction rate of lymphangions. When the transport capacity has been damaged by congenital defect, surgery, trauma, or a mechanical impingement (such as excess belly fat pressing on the inguinal nodes at the groin) this function is impaired. Fluid is left behind in the tissues, causing swelling, as we will see in Chapter 3. The reality that the lymphatic system is *obligated* to remove fluid from tissue is rarely stated. In fact, it doesn't matter what instigated the edema. If any swelling or water retention is present in tissues, this is, in large part, due to a failure of the lymphatic system to remove it.[52]

As the lymphatic system carries out the task of fluid evacuation and transport, it is also performing waste removal. Both noxious and benign particles are discharged from cells and require removal from the tissues to minimize damage. A diet high in inflammatory foods that causes an influx of toxins into the tissues may place undue stress on the lymphatics to perform this function. It becomes particularly important for individuals with a lymphatic disorder to minimize their exposure to toxic foods to lessen the burden on their lymphatic system. The process of discovering individual tolerances for particular foods will be discussed in Chapter 5.

Immune Purpose – Overt Surveillance.

The lymphatic system is part of both the innate and adaptive immune systems. *Innate immunity* is our inborn natural defense and is a broad and non-specific, but fast, response. Our lymphatic system participates in innate immunity by its constant surveillance as fluid passes through the lymph nodes and other lymphoid organs described in the earlier section about lymphatic anatomy. Macrophages in the nodes can kill and digest bacteria along with parasites. Those same macrophages will also secrete cytokines which mobilize other components of the immune system. Removal of lymph nodes, commonly done in the treatment of cancer, can compromise these immune functions of our lymphatic system to such a degree that frequent infections occur in the regions served by the removed nodes.[53]

Even though this nonspecific response of the lymphatic system can occur within hours of a threat entering the body, sometimes it is not fast enough. Specialized white blood cells, called *dendritic cells*, patrol the body for pathogens that they then transport to lymph nodes to be dealt with.[54] If picked up in an outpost of the body not near a node depot, taking the traditional route by entering a lymph capillary can take too long to get to the expressway of a lymph collector or trunk and eventually to a lymph node. In this case, the dendritic cell can take a short cut by entering directly into a larger lymphatic vessel. Usually entry in lymph collectors is much more difficult because of the very tight junctions of the vessel walls, but recent research has shown that under conditions of chronic inflammation, the wall junctions are loosened and allow dendritic cells to slip inside.[55]

Lymphoid organs such as the thymus gland and spleen are involved with *adaptive immune* functions. The adaptive immune system has a slower, but more targeted response to pathogens. The thymus gland develops lymphocytes to directly fight particular invaders. Next, the spleen, among other functions, stores those lymphocytes until needed. When a certain pathogen is recognized, these specialized lymphocytes mount a massive and quite focused attack. These prepared lymphocytes will also multiply rapidly and be ready if this specific pathogen shows up again. Bone marrow, once thought of as solely a place for red blood cell generation, is also highly involved in adaptive immunity. Lymphoid organs are also important for regulating the immune cells and keeping them from attacking our healthy cells. Autoimmune diseases occur when our immune cells stop recognizing the difference between 'self' and 'foreign invader.'

Dietary Fat and Reverse Cholesterol Transport.

With the exception of medium chain triglycerides (MCTs), the lymphatic system is responsible for transporting all dietary fat directly from the intestines to blood circulation. It is truly amazing that dietary fat is so important to our bodies that a system evolved just for conveying that fat to where it is needed. Specialized intestinal lymphatics, called lacteals, absorb dietary fat from the intestinal villi and deliver this fatty fluid, or chyle, to the thoracic duct where it is then transported to the blood circulatory system via the subclavian vein. Approximately 2500 milliliters of chyle per day are transported by the lymphatic system, the flow rate being entirely dependent upon eating or fasting.[56]

Interestingly, the lymphatic system has a much higher concentration of lymphocytes (immune cells) than blood and this is further concentrated in chyle, making up approximately 25 percent of the contents.[56] Loss of dietary fat and lymphocytes, as seen in chyle leaks due to trauma, may have a significant impact on infection frequency.[57] A study by Miura and colleagues in 1987 showed a correlation between the amount of fat eaten and a beneficial increase in the movement of lymphocytes by the lymphatic system. Over ten times the amount of lymphocyte transport was seen after absorption of dietary fat in rats. The authors suggested that there may be an immune system mechanism that prepares and maintains the immune system by movement of lymphocytes in response to fat metabolism.

It may even be true that fat is essential to the proper functioning of the lymphatic system. In Chapter 3, we will discuss evidence that fat fuels the lymphatics, which becomes particularly important when there is a lymphatic impairment. It is disappointing that when there is an impairment to the abdominal lymphatics, the traditional medical and nutritional response has been to limit dietary fat intake to primarily MCTs in an effort to lessen the burden on the intestinal lymphatics and thoracic duct.[58] This may be misguided at best and could be potentially harmful. Limiting fat intake to MCTs can cause a deficiency in essential fatty acids and, startlingly, the lymphatic system will start absorbing MCTs, fatty acids that are almost never found in lymph, in a desperate attempt to get the fats it needs.[30]

Our lymphatics are responsible for carrying another important fat: cholesterol. *Forward cholesterol transport* is the process of bringing cholesterol to the tissues from the liver. Once nutrients are delivered to tissues and utilized, any excess cholesterol not needed by the cells begins its *reverse cholesterol transport* aboard high density lipoproteins (HDL) through the lymphatic system.[59] This very important function of the lymphatic system will be further explored in Chapter 4.

Better imaging has led to an increased awareness of lymphatic system anatomy and its important functions. This, in turn, has led to a better understanding of disorders of the lymphatic system as well as best practices for managing these conditions. In the next chapter, the most common lymphatic disorders and their treatment will be discussed.

Chapter 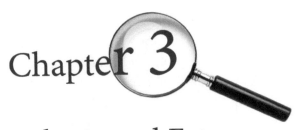 3

Lymphatic and Fat Disorders Explained

"Now, Watson, let us have the facts."
—*Sir Arthur Conan Doyle, The Adventure of the Bruce-Partington Plans*

A lymphatic or fat disorder can have a significant impact on quality of life, particularly if a limb or body part becomes very large or disfigured. For instance, lymphedema in a leg can create difficulties with walking, bathing, or fitting into shoes. A woman with lipedema may suffer from severe pain in her lower body, keeping her from participating fully in family activities. A person with lymphedema in the trunk may experience gastrointestinal distress and difficulty breathing. A woman with breast cancer-related lymphedema in an arm may complain of having to purchase shirts that are several sizes too large just to accommodate the bulk of her swollen arm. The affected region may feel heavy and achy and, if present in an arm or leg, tend to tire more quickly than unaffected limbs. If the swollen body part cannot be disguised by clothing, embarrassment, altered body image, and social discomfort may result. The knowledge that lymphatic and fat disorders are chronic conditions for which there is no cure can lead to despair. All of these scenarios can result in feelings of inadequacy and hopelessness that can foster choices of isolation, less social interaction, and a negative quality of life.

Likewise, it would make sense that improved management of a lymphatic or fat disorder will mean dramatic improvement in quality of life. The first step in successful management of a chronic condition is accurate diagnosis. As we continue to decipher the Lymphatic Code, this chapter will focus on the most prevalent lymphatic disorders, including lymphedema, lipedema, and several other types of edema and their most common treatments.

It is not unusual for several types of swelling to be present in one individual. This may be evident when lipedema and lymphedema occur together. If they do, the condition is sometimes referred to as *lipo-lymphedema*. When both venous and lymphatic disease take place together, the diagnosis is *phlebo-lymphedema*. An example of phlebo-lymphedema is prostate cancer-related lymphedema in a leg that also has *chronic venous insufficiency.*

Lymphedema

Lymphedema is a chronic condition of fluid retention in tissues that presents as gradual swelling of a body part, usually an arm or leg, but lymphedema can occur in any part of the body that has some impairment of the lymphatic system. In the lower body, swelling will usually start at the foot and may eventually encompass the entire leg. In the arm, by comparison, onset is most commonly in the elbow region, with gradual progression both toward the wrist and to the upper arm. Another interesting difference between lymphedema of the leg versus the arm is that the foot is almost always involved when lymphedema develops in the leg, but a person with arm lymphedema may have the hand spared.

Primary lymphedema is a rare hereditary condition in which the lymphatics are poorly formed or non-existent in any region of the body, causing a body part or region to swell due to poor lymphatic drainage. Swelling may be apparent at birth or may not appear until years later. Lymphedema that presents at birth is called *congenital;*

before age 35 is termed *praecox;* and after age 35 is labelled *tardum.* It is important to note that someone with primary lymphedema may have to modify or limit participation in certain tasks or activities, but otherwise should enjoy a normal life expectancy and quality of life. For an excellent video of a young woman telling her story of growing up with primary lymphedema, see the link to Allyson's Story under Resources in Appendix III.

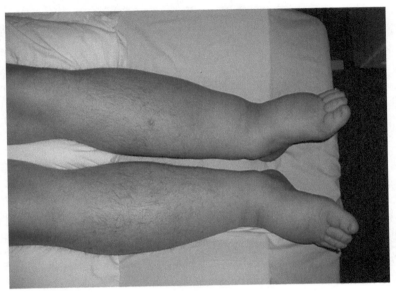

Figure 8. Primary (hereditary) lymphedema in the legs.

Secondary lymphedema is much more common and results from surgery or other trauma that harms the lymphatic system. Worldwide, the most frequent cause of secondary harm to the lymphatic system is a parasitic infection called *filariasis,* though it is primarily limited to tropical and subtropical regions. Poor access to health care, limited education regarding transmission prevention, improper hygiene and skin care all contribute to increased incidence and severity of the condition.

In North America, however, secondary lymphedema is more likely to be diagnosed after treatment for cancer and various other surgeries. Surgical trauma can result in a disruption of lymphatic drainage that leads to swelling in the affected body region. For instance, treatment for breast cancer may involve removal of the affected breast and lymph nodes in the neighboring axilla (underarm). Axillary lymph nodes drain fluid from the adjacent chest, back, and arm. Removal of one or more lymph nodes may cause fluid to build up in any of these areas but, most commonly, fluid builds up in the arm and/or breast.

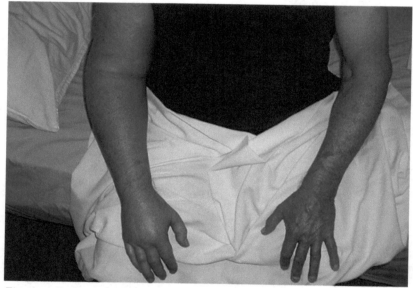

Figure 9. Cancer-related lymphedema of the arm.

With increased understanding of the pathophysiology of lymphedema, we now know that this is an inflammatory condition resulting in *reactive fibrosis* of the skin, underlying subcutaneous tissues, and even the lymphatics themselves.[60] The progressive thickening and hardening of skin and other tissues can restrict movement and cause discomfort. This can also result in increased fluid retention and a higher risk of infection and further scarring in the affected region. Skin can thicken to such a degree that it becomes difficult to pinch the skin at the base of the toes or fingers. This is termed a positive *Stemmer sign*.

Chronic swelling attracts fat causing much of the fluid in a swollen area to be replaced with sometimes quite excessive amounts of fat, seemingly unrelated to whether or not there is an overall weight problem.[61] This fatty tissue will not reduce with conservative treatment measures such as massage or compression therapy, nor is it responsive to traditional low-calorie, low-fat weight loss dieting. For this reason, specialized liposuction techniques were developed to decrease the excessive volume of adipose tissue in a limb with lymphedema.[62] Anecdotally, however, we do see lymphedema fat diminish with a ketogenic diet. Here is one person who had excessive adipose tissue removed prior to adopting a low carbohydrate diet:

> *"By doing research online, I discovered a surgeon in LA who dealt with lymphedema patients. Consequently, I had lymphatic liposuction performed and also a lymph node transfer from my right armpit to my left thigh. Both procedures were very helpful, especially removing 3.5 pounds of adipose tissue from my leg!"*
> —Jean R.

Lymphedema patients often get repeated bouts of cellulitis and other infections, some more frequent than others. Several factors may contribute to a variation in the incidence and severity of infections experienced. One study found gender and location of lymphedema were important: men had more infections than women, and those with lymphedema in the leg versus an arm were more likely to have an infection. Other factors that increased infection risk were low household income and less diligence in lymphedema self-care practices.[63] Infection may also be due to difficulty transporting immune cells to the infection site or removing *antigens* (toxins, bacteria, viruses and other foreign invaders) by a malformed or damaged lymphatic system.[64] However, another cause of infection may be based more in poor nutrition. Malnutrition exponentially increases the risk of infection and infectious disease which can weaken every part of the immune system.[65] Therefore, it becomes imperative for anyone with lymphedema to bolster their immune system with proper nutrition.

It is necessary to also acknowledge the potentially significant psychological impacts of living with a chronic and sometimes disfiguring condition like lymphedema. Although many people lead productive and fulfilling lives with lymphedema, the distress that can be associated with it cannot be ignored. Lymphedema can contribute to negative feelings and psychological distress such as poor body image, lowered self-esteem, sadness, and loss of confidence which all may lead to a feeling of social isolation and a perception of being marginalized in society.[66,67] But in one study, interestingly, the severity of lymphedema did not seem to impact overall quality of life.[68] The authors found that other factors, such as function and pain, were more important for quality of life than the size of their limb.

Although lymphedema is a chronic condition, it can be reduced and managed, even many years after onset, by conservative measures. The gold standard for treatment is Complete Decongestive Therapy (CDT). CDT consists of manual lymph drainage, which is a gentle massage technique that reroutes fluid around an obstruction, compression therapy, decongestive exercises including deep breathing, and meticulous skin care. During the intensive phase of treatment, compression therapy is best provided with specialized short stretch bandages over various padding products to facilitate the evacuation of fluid and reduce fibrosis while protecting the skin and tissue. Optimal treatment during this phase is provided five days per week and could take several weeks depending upon the severity of the lymphedema and the existence of other complicating medical or social conditions.[69]

> *"I had a double mastectomy because I had breast cancer for the second time, 17 years apart. I think they did the surgery with a bulldozer. I didn't heal well...The best and only good thing about my adventure was that it led me to Leslyn Keith. Sweet Mercy! My lymph system was damaged and confused. With her massage, she taught it what direction to travel and taught me how to deal with it."* —Linda P.

After discharge from treatment, lymphedema management transitions to the self-care phase in which a personal protocol for caring for lymphedema long-term is created. This phase may constitute a considerable time investment as well as a significant economic strain for someone with lymphedema.[70] Manual lymph drainage may continue to be performed on a regular basis either by the individual or a caregiver. Compression self-management techniques may include compression garments with varying elasticity and adjustability depending on individual needs, preferences, and abilities. Exercise can be helpful, and recommendations for exercise will be further discussed in Chapter 8. Other modalities which may be employed to augment management of lymphedema in this phase can include vibration, sport taping, and the use of pneumatic compression pumps. Some may opt for a surgical intervention, as microsurgical techniques to remove excess fat tissue, connect lymph vessels to veins, and transplant lymph nodes are continually being improved upon and employed more frequently, sometimes even preventively.[71]

Lipedema

Lipedema is a poorly recognized, chronic, and generally progressive adipose tissue disorder that almost exclusively affects women. It is characterized by a symmetrical enlargement of the lower body due to excessive fatty deposits from waist to ankles, easy bruising, orthostatic edema, and pain. First reported by physicians at the Mayo Clinic in 1940,[72] this condition continues to remain a poorly understood, largely underdiagnosed, and profoundly impactful syndrome.

Although considered by some clinicians to be exclusively an adipose tissue disorder without an edema component,[73] evidence of lymphatic dysfunction associated with lipedema continues to mount. Several imaging studies have shown damaged lymphatics in a significant proportion of women with lipedema, independent of severity of their condition.[74,75,76] In 2017, a research group at Vanderbilt University Medical Center in Nashville, Tennessee, led by Rachelle Crescenzi, found higher levels of sodium and water in the subcutaneous fat in women with lipedema. Several researchers have postulated that lipedema fat traps fluid and becomes waterlogged, effectively overwhelming the lymphatic system. Quite recently, a biomarker for lymphatic impairment, platelet factor 4 (PF4), has been identified. PF4

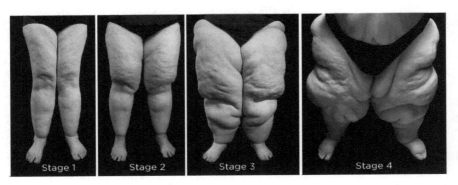

Figure 10. Four Stages of Lipedemia. (Lipedemia Simplified, LLC. 2017-2021. All rights reserved. Used with permission.)

levels were also elevated in lipedema but not in obesity.[61] Hopefully, soon, there will be a diagnostic test to assess PF4 levels in candidates with suspected lymphatic damage.

A common complaint of women with lipedema is pain in the regions of excessive fat deposition. The pain can be so severe that this condition has been called a "painful fat" disorder[77] and may be a significant factor in reduced mobility and quality of life for this population. As many as 89.7 percent of women with lipedema reported daily pain in one study.[78] It is unclear what the source of pain is in lipedema, but many theorize that inflammation is the cause. By removing inflammatory foods from their diets, many women involved in a lipedema Facebook group (see Resources, Appendix III) report that their pain is significantly reduced or completely resolved, sometimes within two weeks of adopting a ketogenic eating plan.

Perhaps the most devastating psychological impact of lipedema is the hopelessness women feel when they are told that treatment options are limited and the condition is generally believed to be non-responsive to diet and exercise. It may be, however, that lipedema is only "non-responsive" to the typical low-calorie, low-fat weight-loss diet. This dietary intervention seems to reduce fat only on the upper body, resulting in further disproportion, poor body image, and increased embarrassment. Anecdotally, on social media groups for women with lipedema engaged in a ketogenic lifestyle, fat loss occurs on the upper and lower body with this way of eating.

The etiology of lipedema remains uncertain. Onset seems to coincide with times of significant sex hormone upheaval, such as during puberty, pregnancy, and menopause. The high frequency of this timing has led many researchers to believe that estrogen is a driver of lipedema, but this theory presents a curious paradox: estrogen levels increase at puberty while they decline sharply at menopause. Another powerful hormone, insulin, may also be acting in lipedema as these landmark events are also normally times of increased insulin resistance. Among the many jobs of insulin are increasing fat storage and reducing fat burning. When our cells become resistant to the signals of insulin, we need more of it to get sugar out of the blood and into fat cells. More insulin means increased buildup of fat tissue. Enter another paradox: typically, women with lipedema have a low incidence of diabetes which is normally associated with insulin resistance. Lastly, it has also been theorized that there is a genetic component due to the strong commonality of body shape between women in a family group, but so far a culpable gene has not been identified.

An examination of human evolution may give us some possible answers. Dr. Paula Stewart, a physician who specializes in the treatment of lymphatic and fat disorders, suggests that women with lipedema may be the Mother of our Species. She proposes that early females who were adept at storing fat on their thighs and buttocks were much more likely to survive famine and to reproduce. Early human statuary is rife with fertility goddesses in the classic lipedema shape (see Figure 11). Dr. Stewart also noticed another amazing detail about women with lipedema when she experimented with using the human chorionic gonadotropin (HCG) diet with this population. This weight-loss regimen combines injections of HCG, a hormone that mimics pregnancy, with a very low-calorie and low-fat diet. She found that women with lipedema were satiated and reported plenty of energy at 500 calories/day, possibly due to a facility for burning lower body fat stores to support pregnancy in times of food scarcity, while non-lipedemic women complained bitterly of constant and tremendous hunger on that same energy input.

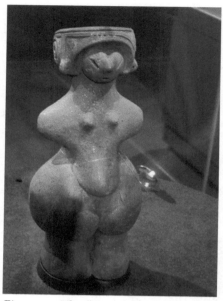

Dr. Caroline Pond, a professor of comparative anatomy with an interest in the evolution of adipose tissue, noted that "thick thighs and large buttocks

Figure 11. The "Jōmon Venus." Ancient Japanese female figurine with small waist and large hips/legs. ([Wikimedia Commons](#))

that enable women to maximize energy reserves without compromising longevity"[19] became sexually more desirable due to their better chance of survival through reproduction and child-rearing during food shortages. The rich localized fat stores in this body shape spectacularly supported lactation as well, supplying an infant with the nourishment crucial for rapid growth. Pond also believes that the large lower body shape was encouraged in females even after their reproductive years concluded, as they had energy reserves that increased life-expectancy and were, thus, then present to perform valuable contributions as grandmothers.[19]

Finally, Pond notes that adaptive obesity is seen in nature, commonly with hibernating animals, to allow for survival without nourishment for months. This is never associated with cardiovascular disease, diabetes, or reproductive dysfunction such as in polycystic ovary syndrome (PCOS). Likewise, women with lipedema have a low incidence of metabolic conditions such as diabetes, until they develop abdominal obesity. This suggests that excessive adipose tissue in the lower body, in itself, may not be metabolically pathological, although it causes orthopedic, hygienic or other symptoms including pain, bruising with minimal trauma, and edema. Although 200,000 years of human evolution brought about genetic modifications for female adaptive obesity, comparatively very little time has elapsed for present-day women with a propensity for lower body fat deposition to possibly adjust to the modern Western diet. While animals and prehistoric females were able to attain adaptive "natural obesity",[19] modern day women with lipedema, through no fault of their own, have developed a painful fat disorder.

Recent estimations show that abdominal obesity co-occurs with lipedema as much as 88 percent of the time,[73,79] significantly complicating the condition. For this reason, various weight loss surgeries and/or liposuction procedures are now commonly considered as a "treatment" for lipedema. While I explain further in Chapter 7 why I believe that bariatric surgery is not an answer for a nutritional failure, let me discuss here why liposuction when not coupled with dietary change won't be the magic bullet that many women with lipedema are hoping it to be. While there are ample reports of a dramatic decrease in pain and limb size for women with lipedema post-liposuction[80,81,82] it is unlikely these changes will be permanent if a high carbohydrate diet is continued.[83] The increased amount of fat needing to be stored when insulin levels are high simply must go somewhere. If you no longer have fat cells on your lower body, it will simply go to other locations which may prove to be cosmetically unpleasant at best and metabolically unhealthy at worse.[84] Nonetheless, combining a ketogenic lifestyle with liposuction for those women suffering with more severe symptoms associated with lipedema may prove to be a valuable treatment option.

Because of its impact on many areas of life, the treatment of lipedema should be holistic to address every psychosocial as well as physical need. See the Lipedema Simplified MasterClass program listed in Resources (Appendix III) for an example of one such program. Treatment by a therapist knowledgeable about lipedema may include manual lymph drainage, skin care, compression therapy, pain management, and nutritional and psychosocial support. If obesity is a comorbidity, weight management should also be provided. Many women with lipedema also employ alternative complementary therapies including dry brushing, vibration, rebounding, Epsom salt baths, and supplements.

Edema

According to the International Society of Lymphology 2020 Consensus Document,[85] an accurate diagnosis of lymphedema is only made when edema results from some sort of impairment of the lymphatic system, whether primary or secondary, causing a reduced capacity of the lymphatic system to transport fluid. Here, we will discuss swelling that occurs in an intact lymphatic system that is simply overwhelmed by an increased fluid load, such as in lower leg swelling that results from congestive heart failure.

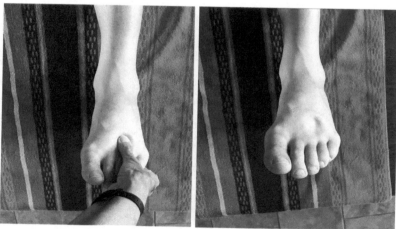

Figure 12. Testing for pitting edema.

The term *edema* is used when fluid overload is the origin of swelling, rather than being the result of some mechanical insufficiency or obstruction to the lymphatic system. Additionally, the composition of fluid in edema is different from that found in lymphedema.

Lymphatic obstruction or impairment causes the fluid in the tissues to become protein-rich, while edema present in an intact system has a much lower protein content.

One way to test for edema, or swelling, is to press the swollen tissue firmly with the pad of the thumb, holding it for at least ten seconds. When pressure is released, an indent in the tissue is a clear indication of the presence of edema (see Figure 12). This is called pitting edema with the severity of pitting usually correlating with the severity of edema.

Injury/Trauma/Post-Surgical.

Swelling is a normal response to injury or trauma and is an initial step in the healing process. Edema due to a broken bone, for instance, creates a natural splint that makes it difficult to move the area. The forced immobility can create a healing environment. This type of edema is also normal when associated with surgery and wound healing. In these instances, the edema should be carefully monitored for infection, and managed to prevent an excessive amount of swelling, but it is generally an expected and non-pathological effect of injury. Management can include complete decongestive therapy with gentle compression dependent on appropriateness and tolerance. A ketogenic diet will reduce inflammation and promote the healing process.

Vascular Impairment.

The most common cause of swelling is due to a vascular impairment called chronic venous insufficiency (CVI). CVI is a problem with veins in the legs due to *venous reflux* (venous blood flows back into the tissues), an obstruction such as a blood clot (deep vein thrombosis or DVT), or a combination of the two reasons. High blood pressure in the leg veins from reflux or an obstruction will result in distended veins and valves that no longer work to keep the venous blood flowing in the proper direction to the heart. One of the biggest risk factors for developing CVI is obesity.[86]

The most common symptoms of CVI are pain, heaviness, swelling and cramps in the lower legs. Later, a dark brown stain will appear on the lower calves, called *hemosiderin staining*. A further complication may be attendant wounds, usually just above the ankles.[87] Treatment involves manual lymph drainage, skin care, and compression therapy. Life-long management will include wearing compression stockings, healthy low-carbohydrate nutrition, and regular exercise. Continued management may also include using a pneumatic pump. In some cases, surgical procedures to close off and/or remove damaged veins may be necessary.

Organ Failure.

Heart, lung, kidney, or liver impairment may result in swelling in the lower legs. Without intervention for the swelling, and with continued worsening of the organ failure, swelling can gradually continue to encompass the entire lower body. Organ failure and the subsequent edema, however, can be managed and may never progress beyond the ankles. Treatment will include medical management of the condition, such as with medications and/or surgery. Similarly to CVI, edema due to organ failure will also be treated with manual lymph drainage, skin care, and compression therapy. A healthy low carbohydrate diet and exercise as tolerated is also recommended.

Nutritional Deficiency.

Illnesses and treatments common to lymphedema patients may result in malnutrition, such as chemotherapy-induced poor appetite or malabsorption of nutrients after weight-loss surgery. In both of these cases, the patient may have been referred for lymphedema therapy due to lower body edema caused by a protein deficiency.[88] *Hypoproteinemia* (low protein levels in the blood) can be caused by chronic blood loss, but can also be a result of malnutrition. Very low levels of protein in the blood are also seen in a rare condition called *protein-losing enteropathy* in which damage to the intestinal lining results in an excessive loss of protein and low blood albumin levels.[89] It is important to treat the nutritional deficiency medically, if necessary, while also treating the swelling with a program of manual lymph drainage, skin care, compression therapy and healthy eating.

Dependency/Immobility.

Being confined to a wheelchair or having a condition that makes movement difficult, increases the risk for leg swelling. Without the deep breathing and muscle contraction that comes with active movement and exercise, the lymphatics are challenged to adequately evacuate fluid against gravity back to the heart. For this reason, it is important to support the lymphatics effectively to optimize lymphatic functioning, and thus tissue health, as much as possible. Treatment may include CDT, elevating the legs, deep breathing exercises and nutritional intervention.

Medication Side Effect.

Many medications have a side effect of water retention or swelling, especially in the legs. Statin medications, for example, are also well-known to disrupt the creation of CoQ_{10} and commonly have a side effect of leg swelling, possibly due to the drugs' effects on kidney function.[90]

Medication can also cause swelling secondary to a nutritional deficiency due to an action of the medication. For instance, common medications for heartburn are histamine antagonists such as Zantac, or proton pump inhibitors such as Prilosec. If taken on a daily basis for an extended period of time, these heartburn medications can reduce much-needed stomach acid and ultimately compromise digestion and absorption of food. Stomach acid is necessary for the breakdown of foods in the gut to make available the most nutrition possible. For clients with diabetes, their insulin and oral diabetes medications can cause intestinal edema.[91] Intestinal edema obstructs the absorption of CoQ_{10}, an exceedingly necessary nutrient for heart health.[92]

Some medications are known to deplete the body of necessary electrolytes. For instance, the pain medication Carbamazepine lowers the body's store of sodium. Although it is counter-intuitive, having too little sodium can result in swelling just like having too much sodium. This will be discussed further in Chapter 6.

Changing to an alternative medication that may have fewer or less severe side effects will be the first consideration in treating medication-caused swelling. Implementing a healthy diet with ketogenic nutrition may also result in a reduction in dosage or discontinuance of certain medications. A ketogenic diet has been found to be effective for mitigating the causes of many conditions, including diabetes and reflux, as discussed above. Adjusting the dosage or stopping any medication must always be done in consultation with a physician, but the surest way to reduce the impact of medication side effects is to no longer have need of it.

Other Lymphatic Disorders

There are many rare lymphatic disorders that result in impaired lymphatic functioning and associated swelling. A partial list of these disorders is described in the table below.

Lymphangioma	Noncancerous, fluid-filled cysts that occur in lymphatic vessels
Lymphangiomatosis	A rare type of tumor which results from an abnormal development of the lymphatic system that consists of widespread lymphangiomas.
Gorham's Disease	A rare bone disorder characterized by bone loss and often associated with abnormal lymph vessel growth, leading to replacement bone with lymphatic vessels where bone used to be.
Lymphangioleiomyomatosis	Abnormal muscle-like cells begin to grow out of control in certain organs or tissues, especially the lungs, lymph nodes, and kidneys.

Lymphangiectasia	A rare pathologic dilation of lymph vessels, often of the intestinal lymphatics.
Microcystic Lymphatic Malformation	Low-flow vascular malformations composed of multiple small cysts, usually affecting deep-lying structures, which makes their treatment even more difficult and complex.
Hennekam Syndrome	A congenital disorder consisting of intestinal lymphangiectasia, facial anomalies, peripheral lymphedema, and stunted growth and intellectual disability.
Waldmann Disease	A rare intestinal disease characterized by dilated intestinal lymph vessels (lacteals) which cause lymph leakage into the small intestine.

Why a Ketogenic Diet is Good for Lymphatics

...ask not what your lymphatic system can do for
you – ask what you can do for your lymphatic system.
With apologies to President John F. Kennedy

As a clinician, I have come to understand that a ketogenic diet that encourages carbohydrate (sugar and starch) restriction and an increased intake of healthy dietary fats is particularly suited to those with lymphatic disorders. Carbohydrates are inflammatory to the lymphatics and can result in both water retention and reduced lymph flow. In a study on mice that were fed a high fructose (carbohydrate) diet, there was as much as a fifty percent reduction in lymph transport capacity due to the detrimental changes in lymphatic vessels resulting in reduced flow.[93] Another research group, who also looked at an animal model of lymphedema, reported in an unpublished observation that a high fructose diet resulted in a weaker lymph vessel contraction that negatively impacted lymph transport.[94]

Are the results the same in humans? David W., a former patient of mine, found success for both his weight and his primary lymphedema with ketogenic nutrition:

"[I] discovered there were clinics that could actually treat people with my lymphatic condition [and] I found a clinic ... near where I live and made an appointment...At my first visit, Leslyn suggested that I try to follow a ketogenic way of eating prior to any treatment for my lymphedema, as I was extremely overweight...I took her advice and...after about 5 or 6 months, I returned to [the clinic and the therapist,] discovered that I had lost 50 pounds and my legs were already smaller." —David W.

An interesting study with breast cancer survivors using a commercial weight loss diet and exercise had unexpected results.[95] They found that although women lost weight on a Nutrisystem® diet, there was no corresponding reduction in the size of their arm affected by lymphedema. This contradicts the outcomes of every other study that examined weight loss and its impact on lymphedema: weight loss had <u>always</u> correlated with limb volume decrease in previous studies. Why was it not the case in this study? It could be that there was reduced lymph drainage due to the high fructose, thus high carbohydrate, content of Nutrisystem® meal replacements. An already damaged lymphatic system was impaired even further by carbohydrate-induced inflammation.

Another possible benefit of limiting carbohydrates may be the inhibition of *mTOR* (mammalian Target of Rapamycin), a protein that helps control several cell functions, including cell growth and survival. Stimulation of mTOR has been implicated in cancer growth and spread.[96] In the last decade, multiple research studies have shown that medication that inhibits mTOR may be promising for treating lymphatic malformations.[97] Because medications are never without side effects, some of which may be intolerable, dietary change may be a preferred strategy for limiting the action of mTOR.[98]

Carbohydrate restriction is not the only advantage of a ketogenic diet for lymphatic disorders, however. There is also evidence that dietary fats both stimulate lymphatic vessel growth and facilitate lymph transport. One animal study showed increased lymphocyte movement through the lymphatics following a high fat meal.[99] An accelerated lymph flow with dietary fat intake was documented by those same researchers who had noted decreased lymph vessel contraction rate and strength with a high fructose diet.[94]

Another former patient of mine, David D., shares the impact of changing to a ketogenic lifestyle on his lymphedema and his well-being:

> *"After nine months, my weight is 346 pounds (a loss of 68 pounds) and I am able to sleep each night between 6-8 hours. I have more energy and I don't fall asleep during the day. I am now remembering things that I learned long ago and I'm applying those skills to my everyday life more often. My blood pressure is down but most importantly, my right leg is now normal, and my left leg is almost there. My skin is much better with less discoloration, smoother skin and no wounds. Even better, I can reach to my feet and can take care of myself without depending on my wife."* —David D

Just as Dr. Watson was indispensable to the success of Sherlock Holmes, both dietary fat and adipose tissue seem vital to the health and functioning of lymphatics. As discussed in Chapter 1, adipose tissue has been closely allied with lymph nodes and other lymphatic system organs throughout our evolutionary development, and the two remain inextricably linked. In animal research for instance, the fat tissue surrounding lymphatic structures will be tenaciously conserved during prolonged fasting, while other body fat stores are used up to nourish the body.[100,101] Interestingly when the fat surrounding lymphatics is removed, it will regenerate much faster than any other body fat.[102] This suggests that fat tissue is so important to the lymphatics, considerable priority is given to its protection.

Why would adipose tissue be so important to the lymphatic system? It has been suggested by some researchers that agents secreted by lymph nodes may influence both the growth and blood supply for local adipose tissue in order to have an easily accessible and ready energy supply for lymphatic system immune functions.[49] Much of the early work examining the interaction between fat and lymphatics has been done by researchers Natasha Harvey in Australia and Caroline Pond with Christine Mattacks in England.[103,49] They all noticed an association between increased adipose tissue deposits in the presence of chronic inflammation and adipose depletion in the face of acute infection and surmised this may be under the direction of the lymphatic system.

The evidence that dietary fat is just as attractive to the lymphatic system as those special energy depots of body fat surrounding lymphatic organs is also mounting, making a ketogenic diet all the more appealing. As discussed in Chapter 1, two independent animal studies concluded that ketone supplementation stimulated the formation of new lymphatic vessels.[29,28] Further, *lymphatic endothelial cells* (the cells that form the lymph vessel wall) will use ketones for energy even in the presence of glucose.[28] A clinical trial currently in progress in Belgium is testing the effectiveness of a ketogenic diet with people who have lymphedema. The researchers expect to conclude the trial in 2023.[104] It is hypothesized that a ketogenic diet, and subsequent increased ketone levels in the body, will stimulate the formation of new lymphatic vessels resulting in improved lymph drainage from a swollen body part. It is likely that an energy source, namely fatty acids and ketones, that has been conserved throughout evolution can still be used by humans to power the lymphatic system.

A ketogenic lifestyle, it seems, is particularly well-designed for someone with a lymphatic or fat disorder, or really anyone who wishes to keep their lymphatics healthy and functioning. In the next chapter we will explore the unique role that lymphatics play in various medical conditions and how a ketogenic diet will support enhanced lymphatic functioning and improved general health.

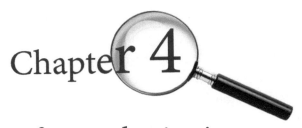

Chapter 4

Role of Lymphatics in Health and Disease

"There are many problems of disease, many strange
pathological possibilities..."
—Sir Arthur Conan Doyle, His Last Bow

As discussed in Chapter 2, the lymphatic system performs several essential functions, including fluid balance/waste removal, immune surveillance, and dietary fat and cholesterol transportation. Despite the indispensability of the lymphatic system, it is still inexplicably viewed, by both the professional and layperson, very simplistically as a passive network of vessels in the body that carries fluid along with various materials from here to there. In fact, the lymphatics may have *the most integral* impact on overall health and disease in *the most basic* way: by being both part of the root cause of disease and part of the resolution for health.

It has been suggested that the wide range of variability seen in a variety of chronic conditions may be due to subtle changes in the lymphatics.[16] According to Dr. Stanley Rockson, a distinguished researcher at Stanford University Center for Lymphatic and Venous Disorders, every organ and system in the body requires healthy lymphatics to function properly, and to such an extent that in the future we may be treating a wide range of diseases by treating the lymphatics.[105]

The central manner of lymphatic system involvement in health and disease is largely through its active participation in the process of inflammation. Inflammation is the body's response to invaders or trauma in that it recruits aid to initiate healing and, as such, is part of a normal healthy process. Acute inflammation calls for an immune response designed to annihilate any toxic materials present. It also simultaneously creates a demand for clearance of debris. The lymphatic system is responsible for both of these jobs. An acute inflammation process is relatively short, lasting anywhere from a few minutes to several days. Signs of acute inflammation include redness, heat, swelling, and pain, which can all be suspiciously similar to signs of infection. It is always wise to have a healthcare provider rule out infection if these symptoms are observed.

Although acute inflammation is completely normal and desirable, problems arise when an inflammatory response turns chronic—a condition which is emerging to be the basis for most modern chronic diseases. When the original irritant or cause of injury lingers for months or years, the body remains in a heightened state of alertness. The continued presence of both toxins and immune cells can cause tissue changes and damage, such as scarring and fibrosis, as well as a long-term sustained need for an immune response. Unfortunately, tissue damage can impair lymph drainage and lead to chronic swelling and increased risk of infection. This harmful cycle of tissue damage and further inflammation needs to be interrupted in order for healing and relief from chronic disease to take place.[465]

Because the lymphatic system plays such an important role in how the human body responds to inflammation, keeping our lymphatics healthy must be a priority. It is well-known that inflammation can induce lymphangiogenesis, or the creation of new lymphatic vessels.[107,108] These new vessels are necessary to bring immune cells where they are needed to kill and dispose of invaders. Such activity will then allow the process of tissue repair to commence. Removal of any excess fluid, waste material, or toxic substances is enhanced with the growth of new lymphatic vessels.

Having extra lymphatic vessels may not always be a good thing, however. If toxic substances are able to slip past immune cells in the lymph nodes, for instance, and are instead efficiently carried to the blood circulatory system via new vessel growth, those invaders are now free to wreak havoc on the rest of the body.[109] Conversely, it has also been shown that new vessel growth associated with inflammation is required for the timely and proper resolution of the inflammatory process. Interruption of lymphangiogenesis can result in prolonged inflammation, aggravation of swelling, and delayed healing.[110] Clearly understanding the interplay between various chronic diseases, inflammation, and the lymphatic system is an important part of the Lymphatic Code. It is my hope that this knowledge will ultimately lead to overall improved health and quality of life for us all.

Cardiovascular Health/Disease

Recent discoveries regarding the role of the lymphatics in health and disease can potentially lead to better outcomes for those with a variety of cardiovascular issues. The essential role of lymphatics was highlighted in a recent discovery that a lack of lymphatics during embryonic development can result in a heart that is as much as a third smaller than normal.[111] Lymphatic impairment may be involved in hypertension (high blood pressure), congestive heart failure (CHF), myocardial infarction (heart attack), venous insufficiency (vein failure), atherosclerosis (sometimes called "hardening of the arteries") and hyperlipidemia (high blood cholesterol).

It has been known for quite some time that the preferred energy sources for the heart, as well as the lymphatic system, are fatty acids and ketone bodies.[112] Although we were temporarily led astray from an appreciation of the health benefits of dietary fats, particularly for the heart, there is now a large body of evidence showing that dietary fat from naturally occurring sources is heart-healthy.[113] In fact, almost all risk factors for heart disease are improved when adopting a well-formulated ketogenic diet that includes plenty of healthy fats.[114]

Hypertension means that the pressure inside blood vessels is elevated, placing an increased force, or pressure, on blood vessel walls. The condition usually starts with a mild injury to blood vessels which then spurs an immune response and inflammation. If the irritant that caused the initial injury continues, chronic inflammation can result, leading to further blood vessel and kidney damage. Each additional injury results in higher blood pressure.[115] The greatest danger from high blood pressure is the potential for a ruptured blood vessel or a blood clot that could lead to damage to organs such as the brain, heart, kidneys, or eyes. People with high blood pressure are at increased risk for stroke, heart attack, and kidney failure.

It is commonly accepted that lifestyle issues such as inactivity, stress, smoking, and diet are major contributors to hypertension, but what part does the lymphatic system play? The immune response to the inflammatory process associated with hypertension has been widely studied,[116] yet the participation of the lymphatic system has rarely been explicitly acknowledged until JE Mekarski published a paper in 1998: *"Hypertension – Essential hypertension is lymphatic: A working hypothesis."*[462] This pioneering paper discussed a direct link specifically with the lymphatic system. Mekarski suggested possible mechanisms for an impaired lymphatic system to increase blood pressure. Several of these mechanisms have since been confirmed through research.[117]

One proposed mechanism – that of the lymphatic system's role in regulating fluid balance in the cardiovascular system – was substantiated in a study by Titze and colleagues in 2009.[118] They described how sodium is sequestered just under the skin inside lymphatic vessels, lessening the effect, they theorized, of sodium in the blood to keep blood pressure lower yet keeping it available as an extremely effective front line defense against infection. Another role of the lymphatic system in hypertension stems from the influence of lymphatics on tissue pressure, and thus on blood pressure, by managing fluid balance. Increased pressure in bodily tissues from fluid congestion can cause a rise in blood pressure. Because the overwhelming majority of fluid and material is removed from tissues by the lymphatics, an impaired or overwhelmed lymphatic system can contribute to hypertension.[118]

The effectiveness of a ketogenic diet for lowering blood pressure has been affirmed in multiple research studies.[119-121] Combined with what we are learning about the beneficial effects of a ketogenic diet on lymphatic health, the best strategy for successfully managing hypertension may be limiting carbohydrate intake and eating plenty of healthy fats.

A **myocardial infarction (MI)**, or heart attack, occurs when a coronary artery (blood vessel in the heart) becomes blocked and a portion of the heart becomes deprived of oxygen and nutrients. An MI can be both painful and scary, as well as confusing, partly because symptoms can be vastly different for each person. Typical symptoms such as chest pain and shortness of breath can make a potential diagnosis of a heart attack more obvious, but many people present with symptoms that are more subtle and baffling. Women may not have any chest pain at all and may instead complain of nausea, jaw pain, or acid reflux.[122]

Within thirty minutes of a heart attack, the lymphatics are called to action to evacuate fluid, proteins, enzymes, and inflammatory agents that have been released in response to an obstruction in a coronary artery, with lymphatic flow rates increasing by as much as fifty percent.[123] Even with this assistance, fluid starts to build up around the heart, making it more difficult to supply oxygen to the heart cells. The accumulation of fluid and toxic substances which now surround the heart causes further damage to the imperiled organ. Medications such as hyaluronidase have been shown to beneficially increase cardiac lymph flow if they are administered within 6 hours of onset of chest pains.[124,125]

As discussed in Chapter 1, the lymphatic system develops unique attributes and properties that can be organ-specific. The heart has its own special lymphatics that are essential for heart health and recovery from heart attack.[126] One study noted a profound increase in cardiac lymph vessel formation in response to heart attack and the administration of an agent that stimulates lymph vessel growth (VEGF-C) further improved heart function.[127] As researchers Veronique Angeli and Natasha Harvey (2015) have said, clearly the lymphatic system is "at the heart of the matter."[22]

Congestive heart failure (CHF) is a chronic weakness of the heart that prevents this vital organ from functioning as well as it should. The most common symptoms of CHF are shortness of breath with minimal exertion, leg swelling, fatigue and an increased heartbeat. Cardiologists would refer patients diagnosed with CHF to my lymphedema clinic for treatment of their leg swelling, but because of the diminished functioning of the heart, these patients were also experiencing increased fluid load in the lungs and surrounding trunk. This meant that they would routinely be out of breath just by walking into the clinic from their car, a distance of less than 200 feet, or getting dressed after their treatment.

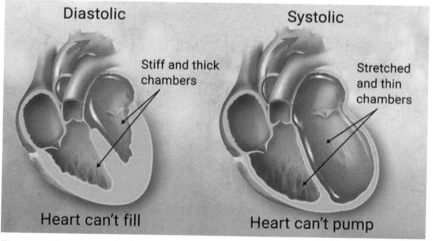

Figure 13. Damage to the heart with Congestive Heart Failure can be from either its inability to fill properly or pump blood adequately.

Frequently reported causes of CHF include hypertension, myocardial infarction (both discussed above), thyroid and kidney disease, diabetes, birth defects, infections, and lifestyle. Lifestyle factors suggested by mainstream medicine are limited to lack of exercise and alcohol/drug abuse and make no mention of diet except for an admonition to reduce salt intake. I believe that all of the noted causes of CHF, with birth defects being the only exception, are actually lifestyle-induced largely due to an inferior diet. It may be that a well-formulated ketogenic diet, with careful monitoring by a cardiologist versed in ketogenic nutrition, can better manage and even greatly improve the symptoms of CHF.[128] It is horrifyingly ironic, then, that the generally accepted diet recommendations encouraged by mainstream medical practitioners to treat CHF likely cause further deterioration to the heart: low sodium, high carb, and low fat.[129]

Mention of the lymphatic system related to CHF has primarily been limited to managing the body's fluid balance related to leg swelling and to water retention in general, especially in the lungs. Usual treatment consists of diuretics (water pills) and other medications, compression stockings, and limiting water and salt intake. Patients are carefully monitored for sudden weight gain as this may indicate increased fluid retention and further compromised health. Typical lymphedema therapy, including manual lymph drainage and compression therapy, is performed with caution to avoid sending too much fluid too quickly out of the legs and towards an impaired heart. One cardiologist said to me that she would prefer that fluid was retained in the legs rather than in the lungs or around the heart.

In the last ten years, an expanded definition of CHF has been called for that places more importance on lymphatics.[130] Philip Houck, a cardiologist and associate professor of medicine at Texas A&M University, is particularly interested in the role of lymphatics in heart failure. He suggests that inflammation, and the response of the lymphatic system, is central to CHF. In fact, comorbidities such as lymphatic dysfunction can worsen the condition and focus should be placed on improving the health of the lymphatic system.[131]

In **chronic venous insufficiency (CVI)**, blood collects in the lower legs when the veins are unable to fight the force of gravity to carry blood back to the heart, largely due to failure of the one-way valves to function properly. As more and more blood pools in the lower legs, the lymphatics quickly become overwhelmed. The inability of the lymphatics to keep up with the increased fluid load then results in swelling. In this way, the failure of the lymphatic system is just as important as venous failure and must be a consideration for treatment of CVI.[132]

At first, swelling may be present just in the ankles and only late in the day, usually completely reducing overnight. Gradually, as the veins become less competent and the lymphatic system becomes more overburdened, swelling will progress to the knees and will only partially resolve with elevation overnight. Later, edema is present in the entire legs and no longer reduces at all with elevation. Mild to severe skin and tissue changes will occur. These include itching, flaking skin, a red or purplish stain on the lower calves, and shallow, poorly healing wounds, usually found just above the ankle.

The most commonly cited reasons for the initial vein impairment in CVI is decreased activity. Less movement means less calf muscle contractions that may eventually result in blood clots and calf muscle weakness. Less common causes of CVI are pelvic tumors and vascular malformations. Recent literature notes not only a higher incidence of CVI when diabetes is also present,[133] but also increased risk of lymphatic failure with diabetes,[45] indicating that diabetes is a risk factor for developing both venous and lymphatic impairment.

Important aspects of treatment for CVI include compression therapy, such as compression wraps, stockings, and/or a pneumatic pump, in conjunction with an exercise program that stimulates the calf muscle pump. Because of the known risk that diabetes poses to blood and lymph vessels, management of venous and lymphatic impairment through a well-formulated low carbohydrate ketogenic diet should be considered first and be part of the overall program for optimal outcomes.[134]

Atherosclerosis is a chronic inflammatory condition, occurring when there is a build-up of fatty plaques in the walls of arteries, most commonly the coronary arteries in the heart. Because the plaques cause the arterial walls to become thickened and stiff, atherosclerosis has been called "hardening of the arteries." In order to function properly, blood vessels need to be flexible and elastic. Hardened and stiff arteries become narrower and are less able to bring nutrients and oxygen to the tissues they serve. This vessel deformity can lead to serious health conditions including heart attack, stroke, hypertension, kidney failure, and blood clots.

Several researchers have correlated lymphatic system impairment with the onset and progression of atherosclerosis.[135,136] Large to medium size arteries have their own lymphatics (lymphatic vasa vasorum discussed below) that may be used to remove inflammatory toxins, transport immune cells, and remove excess cholesterol.[137] Thickening of the arterial wall was observed when lymphatic drainage from the vessel was blocked, so it was surmised that this thickening was due to edema in the vessel wall.[138] There is also an interesting theory that a more dense lymphatic network associated with an artery may actually be protective against atherosclerosis.[139] Thus, facilitating lymphatic growth and drainage may be one important intervention in this disease.

Hyperlipidemia is an abnormally high amount of lipids (fats) in the blood. Although it is not very helpful or descriptive, this condition is also termed *high cholesterol*. The conventional wisdom states that hyperlipidemia is the main cause of atherosclerosis, but this has been strongly questioned of late. Essentially, this popularly accepted theory is that the inside of an arterial blood vessel is damaged, allowing lipoprotein particles (which carry essential cholesterol) to get trapped in the arterial wall, which then leads to plaque formation and ultimately atherosclerosis.

Vladimir Subbotin, a physician, pathologist, and scientist in Russia, does not agree with this theory at all. He demonstrates through imaging that it is more likely that the cholesterol-laden lipoproteins are getting into the vessel wall by way of the <u>outside</u> of the vessel, not from the <u>inside</u>, using specialized minute blood vessels, called *vasa vasorum*. The vasa vasorum are blood vessels that feed the larger arteries.[140] Vasa vasorum are designed to be very leaky vessels and they can easily deliver the large particles of LDL into the outside of the vessel wall. His theory is supported by imaging showing that LDL particles in the vessel wall are more concentrated the closer they are to the outside of the vessel wall and are not seen at all near the inside of the vessel wall until arterial disease is more advanced.

Superior imaging now conclusively demonstrates the presence of a *lymphatic vasa vasorum* that also serves the larger blood vessels and coronary arteries and is intimately involved in arterial health.[141] The lymphatic vasa vasorum is needed for reverse cholesterol transport, that is, removal of excess cholesterol (lipoproteins), from the vessel wall as first described in Chapter 2. It is conjecture at this point, but it may be that when a vein, which lacks a lymphatic vasa vasorum, is used to do the work of a coronary artery, such as in the case in a coronary artery bypass surgery, the newly transplanted vessel may be at a serious disadvantage. The absence of a vasa vasorum may be problematic and allow excess lipoproteins to accumulate. Researchers have looked for the presence of something as the root of heart disease when it in actuality may be a lack: namely proper cardiac lymphatics including the lymphatic vasa vasorum.

Let's take a moment to revisit one of the functions of the lymphatic system in this discussion of hyperlipidemia: reverse cholesterol transport. Cholesterol is needed for many important functions such as producing sex hormones and vitamin D, synthesizing bile, and building cell walls. The human body is adept at making most of the cholesterol it needs, so eating high cholesterol foods does not necessarily increase cholesterol levels in the blood. Normally, the body reduces cholesterol production as dietary cholesterol consumption increases.

Several researchers have found that lymphatics play a very active role in the concentration of high density lipoproteins (HDL) in tissues and lymph fluid, depending on need. The concentration of HDL is generally much higher in bodily tissues and lymph as compared to blood.[142,143] Effective removal of excess cholesterol and triglycerides from tissues becomes critical when lymphatic impairment exists as the evacuation is no longer performed at optimal levels.[144] This concern can be addressed, at least in part, by reducing triglyceride levels in the body through dietary change (see sidebar explanation below).

Carbohydrates and Triglyceride Levels

When we eat carbohydrates, our blood sugar increases in the form of glucose. Much of the glucose is absorbed into our muscles (as much as 80 percent) and is stored there as glycogen.[145] The remainder is stored as glycogen in the liver, but both muscle and liver glycogen storage is limited to approximately one day's worth of energy. Any excess dietary glucose will be packaged into triglycerides which are then released into the bloodstream to be sent to adipose tissue.[146] Fat cells will take in this energy until they, too, cannot accept any more energy. The excess triglycerides are then shunted through lymph vessels as part of the reverse cholesterol transport system back into the bloodstream until eventually the excess triglycerides must be stored in and around organs. This is considered ectopic fat storage and is dangerous to health because it is fat that is stored in an inappropriate place. This is the beginning of fatty liver disease, fatty kidney disease and other fatty organ diseases.

Metabolic Syndrome

After studying diabetes for many decades, respected endocrinologist Dr. Gerald Reaven noted a group of five symptoms that he found to be indicative of future disease. These are abdominal obesity, high blood pressure, high blood sugar, high triglycerides, and low HDL. By definition, if a person has any three of these characteristics, they are said to have metabolic syndrome. Dr. Reaven came to understand that this diagnosis is associated with a significantly raised risk of cardiovascular disease as well as diabetes. Metabolic syndrome is now considered to be the most serious of all global epidemics.[147] Most importantly, for anyone who wants to control and even resolve the symptoms of metabolic syndrome, dietary carbohydrate restriction has been found to be the best means to do so.[148]

Researchers have recently begun to consider not only the effects of metabolic syndrome on the lymphatic system but also how the lymphatic system can contribute to metabolic syndrome.[149] It seems that the unfavorable environment created by metabolic syndrome causes lymphatic vessels to be less efficient at removing inflammatory materials and excess lipoproteins from tissues. A build-up of toxic material creates more inflammation, further harming lymphatics and causing increased deposition of pathological fat tissue. There is now agreement that the damage is bidirectional, with lymphatics being impaired by metabolic syndrome while simultaneously exacerbating the condition.[150,94] Once again, it seems that improving the health of the lymphatic system may have important implications for managing or preventing metabolic syndrome.

Diabetes

Diabetes is a disease in which the body's ability to produce or, in the case of type 2 diabetes, respond to, the hormone insulin is impaired, resulting in abnormal metabolism of carbohydrates and elevated levels of glucose in the blood and urine. In type 1 diabetes, the pancreas stops producing, or doesn't produce enough, insulin. Conversely, in type 2 diabetes, the pancreas produces adequate levels (or in the later stages of the disease, excessively high amounts) of insulin but the body's cells are slow to respond to it. Gradually, the body requires higher and higher insulin levels to remove glucose from the blood. Simply put: people with diabetes have a poor tolerance for foods that metabolize into glucose (carbohydrates). Several studies in the past decade have shown that people with diabetes who adopt a ketogenic diet are able to dramatically decrease or even discontinue insulin therapy altogether.[151,134,152]

It has become increasingly clear that hyperinsulinemia (very high levels of insulin in the blood) can impair lymphatic system function to such a degree that an inadequate immune response can leave the body vulnerable to inflammation and infection.[466,137] Additionally, clinicians have noticed for decades that treatment with insulin induces leg swelling, but the mechanisms have only recently been described. Edema may result from sodium and water retention due to the action of insulin on kidneys and/or pathologically dilated and leaky blood vessels.[153] Research in Joshua Scallan's laboratory at the University of Missouri found an additional lymphatic-related mechanism for swelling associated with diabetes. They showed that mice with type 2 diabetes developed leaky lymphatic vessels due to impairment of nitrous oxide signaling.[45] The frequent episodes of *hyperglycemia*, or high blood sugar, that can be present in diabetes has also been shown to inflame lymphatic vessel walls and increase their leakiness.[154] Because reducing exposure to sugar and starch is most likely beneficial to lymphatic vessel integrity and function, it seems that a ketogenic diet is not only suited to remediating type 2 diabetes but is particularly helpful for repairing the leaky lymphatic vessels that have been impaired by the disease.

Cancer

The spread and progression of cancer is perhaps the most studied context for the lymphatic system. Professor Thomas Seyfried, indefatigable researcher and cancer biologist at Boston College in Massachusetts, states that because cancer cells share characteristics with macrophages (immune cells that roam the lymphatic system looking for invaders), they are also given free reign within the lymphatic system.[155]

There has been a belief for most of the last century that the lymphatic system is a conduit for cancer cells to travel to other parts of the body and thus this system is key in cancer metastasis.[156] The idea is seemingly supported when cancer cells are discovered in the lymph nodes that are draining a tumor. Removal of most, if not all, regional lymph nodes was thought to make metastasis less likely, thus improving survival rates. Unfortunately, although considered life-saving, the practice of removing as many lymph nodes as possible only led to a greater risk of developing lymphedema. New evidence in the last twenty years has not shown that excessive lymph node removal will improve a cancer patient's prognosis, especially in breast cancer and melanoma. Surgeons now take a much smaller sampling of lymph nodes, called a *sentinel lymph node biopsy*,[157,158] resulting in fewer cases of lymphedema.

Another possible method of lymphatic system participation in cancer metastasis may be excessive lymphangiogenesis, the formation of new lymphatic vessels. One study found a poorer prognosis when a tumor is able to recruit a dense lymphatic network.[159] It has been suggested that excessive lymph vessel growth associated with colon cancer is a biomarker for the severity of the disease. The authors even propose that blocking lymph vessel growth should be a target of chemotherapy.[160]

However, more recent research has supported an opposing viewpoint. Several studies have shown that in some cancers, including colorectal cancer, lymphatic vessel proliferation appears to aid the immune response and repress cancer growth.[161,162] It has even been suggested that an enhanced lymphatic system may actually block spreading of a tumor to distant sites.[163] A poorly functioning lymphatic system may be one of the avenues that allows cancer to take hold.[164] Researcher Guillermo Oliver states that a careful balance between encouraging tumor decline rather than tumor growth through lymphatic health needs to be achieved.[16] Clearly, more research is needed to examine the role of the lymphatic system in various cancers and how to use this knowledge to best support successful cancer treatment.

We know from the Warburg Effect that many cancers are glucose-dependent due to the inability of the cancer cell mitochondria, the powerhouse of the cell, to use fat as energy.[165] A ketogenic diet, with sufficient carbohydrate restriction, has been shown to enhance conventional therapies for breast, lung, colon, and brain cancers.[166] Professor Seyfried has commented, "*Simultaneous targeting of glucose and glutamine will kill metastatic cells in the lymphatic system*".[155] A well-formulated ketogenic diet seems particularly suited for cancer-related lymphedema because of its anti-cancer properties along with its enhancement of lymphatic performance.

Respiratory Diseases

The respiratory system is made up of all of the structures that bring air into the body, such as the nose, throat, bronchi, and lungs. Because of the constant need to breathe every minute of every day, any disruption or difficulty with the respiratory system can lead to significant decline in health and well-being. Some of the most common lung illnesses include chronic obstructive pulmonary disease (COPD), emphysema, lung cancer, pneumonia, pleural effusion, and pulmonary fibrosis.

While we know that healthy pulmonary lymphatics are vital for preparing the lungs of a fetus for its first breath as a newborn,[167] these specialized lymphatics also play a critical role in chronic lung conditions.[168] In the case of pulmonary fibrosis, for instance, a greater severity in mediastinal lymph node enlargement (lymph nodes found in the center of the chest between the lungs) indicates a poorer overall prognosis.[169,170] Tuberculosis, another lung disease, may actually be a chronic infection in the pulmonary lymphatics.[171] And in a study on dogs, it was observed that pulmonary lymphatics gradually expanded over time in order to compensate for and help manage chronic pulmonary edema.[172] One reason for the success of lymphatic compensation in compromised lungs may be due to its much greater ability than the blood to absorb debris, particles, and fluid from the lungs.[173]

One method of targeting the lymphatics in the treatment of respiratory illness is through breathing exercises. As we have seen in Chapter 2, breathing is an effective means for activating the contraction of lymphatic vessels and increasing lymph flow which promotes lung health. Breathing exercises that coordinate deep slow breathing through the nose in conjunction with contraction of the key trunk muscles including the diaphragm, abdominal, pelvic floor, and intercostal muscles may be the most effective in facilitating improved lymphatic function and restoring respiratory health. Suggested breathing exercises will be described in Chapter 8.

The *respiratory quotient (RQ)*, or the ratio of carbon dioxide produced to oxygen consumed, is a common marker of respiratory health, with lower values associated with better health and higher values correlated with increased work for the lungs. The RQ from the metabolism of carbohydrate is highest at 1.0 and lowest with fat at 0.7. Thus, eating carbohydrates produces more carbon dioxide and creates more respiratory stress,[174] suggesting that a low–carbohydrate ketogenic diet should have a positive impact on respiratory function. Indeed, healthy adults tended to perform better with either glycogen store depletion or consuming a high fat diet, since both options required fat to be used for fuel.[175,176]

A well-formulated ketogenic diet seems particularly beneficial for respiratory illness for this reason. In one study, patients with COPD adhering to a low-carbohydrate high-fat diet had significantly better RQ, as well as other indicators of improved respiration, compared to the standard high carbohydrate diet group.[174] Other research has shown the beneficial impact of a ketogenic diet on both a viral influenza infection and respiratory failure requiring ventilation.[177,178] Kelly Bell, who suffers from infiltration of a polymer to his lymphatic duct and compromised lungs, relates how a ketogenic diet improved his breathing almost immediately:

> *"Within the first week [of starting keto], I lost over 9 pounds and felt like I could finally take a deep breath. I went for an evening one-mile walk and ended up walking three miles for the first time in years. In the first month, I lost over 33 pounds and knew I no longer needed supplemental oxygen." —Kelly B.*

Lastly, a ketogenic diet increases levels of leptin in the body.[179] Leptin is a hormone that, among other functions, suppresses appetite, strengthens immune function, and stimulates respiration.[180] The positive effect of leptin on various respiratory diseases, such as asthma, COPD and lung cancer, is well documented.[181] Additionally, lung development and maturation is supported by leptin. All of these properties of leptin suggest that the elevated levels present with a ketogenic diet would support lymphatic function and be favorable for addressing respiratory illnesses.

Neurodegenerative Diseases

Conditions that primarily involve damage or decay of neurons, or nerve cells, in the brain are classified as neurodegenerative diseases. Because neurons do not normally reproduce, damaged neurons are not replaced, making most neurodegenerative diseases progressively debilitating, with gradually worsening disorders in movement, altered sensation, and/or hampered cognition. The two most common neurodegenerative diseases are Alzheimer's disease and Parkinson's disease. Multiple Sclerosis is a neurodegenerative disease that is also considered an autoimmune disease and will be discussed in a later section of this chapter.

A recent exciting breakthrough in the field of lymphology is that of the brain lymphatics, or glymphatics, and their special role in brain functioning and health. This important discovery came out of neuroscientist Jonathan Kipnis' lab at the University of Virginia School of Medicine. The 2015 paper authored by Kipnis and postdoctoral fellow Antoine Louveau described how the glymphatics are involved in central nervous system waste removal, transport of glucose and fat in the brain, regulation of the interchange and removal of cerebrospinal fluid (the fluid that bathes the brain and spinal cord), as well as important immune functions.[37] Prior to the discovery of the glymphatics, there were several theories as to why the brain might be resistant to infection. The main assumption was the inability of most pathogens to cross the blood-brain barrier. Now it is believed that the specialized central nervous system glymphatics form an additional barrier to infection.[37,182] This was confirmed by a recent study that showed that brain lymphatic fluid contains significantly more metabolites than does cerebrospinal fluid, demonstrating the much stronger role of glymphatics in removing noxious pathogens from the brain.[183]

Although there was some inkling about the presence of lymphatics in the brain prior to their 2014 discovery, it took some time before adequate imaging techniques could be developed to allow them to be visualized, as they are generally in a collapsed state while we are awake. They become much more active during sleep. Once enhanced imaging was developed, it was clear that the lymphatics in the brain showed similar features in both form and function with lymphatics in the rest of the body. Brain lymphatics actually perform a job previously thought to be carried out chiefly by cerebrospinal fluid.[184] These brain lymphatics are a "clearance route" for the brain, moving debris alongside arteries, veins, and nerves to the lymph nodes in the neck.[185]

Although the brain comprises just two percent of the body's total weight, it requires twenty percent of all of the cholesterol utilized by the body.[186] Itself composed of sixty percent fat, the brain depends upon cholesterol for proper development and adult function. Cholesterol is literally "food for thought" as its depletion in the brain is known to lead to neurodegenerative disease.[187] Unlike the rest of the body which is supplied with cholesterol from the liver, the brain has the ability to make all of its own needed cholesterol. The highway for fat and cholesterol distribution in the brain is the glymphatics.[188]

What might encourage the flow of lymph within the brain? It is theorized that it is pressure from the constant production of cerebrospinal fluid, breathing (particularly deep breathing), and pulsation of adjacent arteries.[188] Most influential in glymphatic activity, however, is the increased space available between cells with the brain cell shrinkage that occurs during sleep or anesthesia. In fact, when the brain is awake and aware, brain cells expand so much that the glymphatic activity can be reduced by as much as ninety percent.[189] Hence, a lack of adequate sleeping time could be a possible trigger for many neurological conditions due to the inability of the glymphatics to adequately remove waste and toxins during the prime time of sleep.[189,188] It should be no surprise that a common hallmark of neurodegenerative disorders is an abnormal accumulation of unwanted and potentially noxious metabolites in the brain[190] as well as a high correlation with sleep disturbances.[191]

Alzheimer's disease is a progressive brain disease that is characterized by specific changes in the brain, including amyloid plaques and neurofibrillary tangles that result in a loss of neurons. It is now also referred to as Type 3 diabetes because of the carbohydrate intolerance, insulin resistance, chronic oxidative stress and cognitive impairment seen in this population.[192] Research has shown as well that there is an impaired ability of the brain to use glucose in those with Alzheimer's disease.[193] Additionally, failure of the glymphatics to clear waste, particularly the amyloid plaques, is pivotal in this condition. Proper glymphatic functioning may be a necessary requirement for proper cognitive function.[190]

Making lifestyle changes that would benefit the glymphatics as well as the brain insulin resistance seen in Alzheimer's disease may have a positive impact on this population. Adoption of a ketogenic diet was seen in one study to increase cognition scores significantly in patients with early-stage Alzheimer's disease.[194] Several studies seem to point to not only the benefit of carbohydrate restriction, but also the potential neuroprotective attributes of consuming healthy fats for people with Alzheimer's disease.[195,196,197] Geriatrics researcher Mark Reger in Seattle, Washington wanted to learn whether ketones could be used as an alternative to glucose for energy in the brain for patients with Alzheimer's. Twenty participants with Alzheimer's disease were given a medium chain triglyceride (MCT) drink or a placebo drink. MCTs are a type of fat that is quickly metabolized for energy. Cognition tests given 90 minutes after the drink showed a high correlation between ketone levels and increased cognitive ability. Another study repeated this protocol with twenty Japanese patients and found similar results.[197] Yet another study compared a carbohydrate-restricted diet with a high carbohydrate diet and again found superior improvements in blood panel numbers, weight loss, and memory performance to be associated with higher ketone levels.[198]

Because of the high incidence of sleep disorders in the Alzheimer's disease population, improving sleep hygiene may also have benefits. Most commonly seen disorders are breathing problems (sleep apnea) and restless legs syndrome and are often present in the early stages of the disease or even prior to onset of the condition.[191] Swift diagnosis and treatment of these conditions will enhance the ability to get rejuvenating sleep, which is associated with memory improvement.[199] Intriguing research using animals has suggested that sleeping on one's side appears to facilitate glymphatic brain drainage the best.[200]

Parkinson's disease is a progressive neurodegenerative disease marked by tremors, rigidity, a shuffling gait, and, at later stages, cognitive impairment. The accumulation of Lewy bodies and a misfolded protein called alpha-synuclein in the brain as well as a deficiency in the neurotransmitter dopamine causes gradual damage and deterioration.[201,184] As with Alzheimer's disease, failure of the glymphatics to remove noxious materials allows the condition to worsen.

Impaired brain lymphatics is not the only lymphatic failure evident in Parkinson's disease. In a case study report from a hospital in Zurich, Switzerland, a woman with Parkinson's disease and lower leg swelling is discussed.[202] Although the authors acknowledge that the main culprit of her edema may be a reduced calf muscle pump due to the shuffling gait characteristic of Parkinson's, they also report a pressure increase in the tissues and lymph capillaries of the lower leg that they believe contributed to the problem. Also, in a study that followed Parkinson's disease patients over twenty years (five years prior to diagnosis through fifteen years after diagnosis), this group was almost twice as likely to have a lymphatic or venous condition as their healthy counterparts.[203] This was consistent with my own clinical experience in which I was asked to collaborate with a neurologist's Parkinson's disease practice due to the high incidence of leg swelling the doctor had witnessed in his patients.

In my own practice, I observed reduced weight and decreased leg swelling in patients with Parkinson's disease who adopted a ketogenic diet. Furthermore, medical literature points to some possible modifications that can be made to a ketogenic diet to make it more effective for treatment of Parkinson's disease. While a low-protein diet improves the bioavailability of Levodopa (a common drug used to elevate dopamine levels in people with Parkinson's), this may not be favorable for an elderly population who may suffer from muscle loss and have higher protein needs.[204] Therefore, it may be best to adjust protein content according to need, along with consultation with a medical provider.

Another modification to a ketogenic diet that may be useful for this population is increasing saturated fat and decreasing polyunsaturated fat intakes. In a study examining the impact of various fatty acids on Parkinson's disease, it was found that the accumulation of alpha-synuclein (the misfolded protein inadequately cleared by glymphatics) was increased by the consumption of excessive polyunsaturated fatty acids. A diet high in monounsaturated fatty acids had no such effect, and saturated fatty acid intake actually reduced alpha-synuclein levels.[205]

Research has shown a ketogenic diet to be of benefit in Parkinson's disease, even if the diet is not formulated optimally.[204,206] It seems the diet's restriction of inflammatory carbohydrates in combination with the inclusion of healthy fats is proving to be neuroprotective. In one study, participants completed a randomized trial that compared the effect of a low-fat diet versus a ketogenic diet on their symptoms.[206] Both diet groups did well and showed improvements, but the ketogenic diet group showed much better improvements in nonmotor symptoms such as pain, fatigue and daytime sleepiness, along with cognition. A group of researchers at the Movement Disorders Clinic of Beth Israel Medical Center, led by Theodore B. VanItallie, performed a small pilot study with five patients with Parkinson's using what they termed a "hyperketogenic" diet.[207] Despite the fact that researchers encouraged the subjects to choose polyunsaturated fats over saturated fats (a choice that encourages inflammation), the participants all improved in cognition, activities of daily living, and motor function. The modest so-called "adverse" effects over the 28-day study included weight loss and a need to reduce Levodopa dosage due to feeling "over-medicated."

Gastrointestinal Diseases

The gastrointestinal tract and the lymphatics interact closely throughout the process of digestion. These two major body systems join and cooperate starting with the tonsils, specialized lymphoid organs that monitor food and drink as it enters the body, all the way to the intestinal lacteals, lymphatic capillaries that absorb fats from the small intestine. Lymphatics regulate fluid to the salivary glands, work in the mucosal layers of the stomach, and are involved with the functioning of other digestive organs such as the pancreas, gallbladder, and liver.[208] It is no wonder then, with such a collaboration from beginning to end, that lymphatics play an important role in gastrointestinal health and disease.

The gut is the body's largest interface with the outside world, making the immune surveillance work of the lymphatic system quite demanding. As described in Chapter 2, this work is done primarily with Peyer's patches, aggregated lymphoid nodules that detect need and initiate immune system responses. It is not surprising therefore, that research has unveiled the role of lymphatics in many gastrointestinal disorders including irritable bowel syndrome, pancreatitis, protein-losing enteropathy, Whipple's disease, ascites, Sjogren's disease, and cirrhosis.[208-211] The primary mechanism in these and many other maladies is thought to operate either through poorly formed lymphatics (which allows fluid to accumulate, prevents delivery of nutrients, or upsets the immune system) or by inflammation-caused destruction to both the lymphatics and gastrointestinal system.[208] It appears to be a two-way street between the digestive tract and lymphatics, with impairment in either system causing debilitating dysfunction in the other, both eventually leading to poor metabolic health.[212]

Crohn's disease is chronic inflammation of the digestive tract that can result in ulcers (sores) and fistulae (tunnels) in the intestines. Sufferers can experience abdominal pain, severe diarrhea and fatigue as well as weight loss from malnutrition. Early study of the bowel in people suffering from Crohn's disease showed dramatic changes in the intestinal lymphatics. Although the cause of the disease, or the role of lymphatics in it, was unknown at the time, the abnormal lymphatics were clearly evident. Namely, the affected lymphatics were markedly enlarged, distended and irregularly shaped,"[213] and were associated with abdominal lymphedema.[214] A more recent study found abdominal lymphatic abnormalities in all surveyed patients with Crohn's disease.[215]

As with other conditions, inflammation triggers lymphangiogenesis in Crohn's disease. Even with the presence of more vessels, however, lymph drainage is impaired and inflammatory materials collect around the intestines. Animal studies have shown that this may be due to the faulty pumping of the lymphatic vessels associated with Crohn's.[215] Poor drainage leaves increased levels of harmful bacteria and immune cells in the tissue which in turn increases inflammation.

In a 1979 study of 35 patients with Crohn's disease, it was found that this population consumed a substantially greater amount of sugar and starch, yet equivalent amounts of protein and fat, compared to controls. This dietary pattern seemed to be long-standing and was followed well before the onset of any symptoms of Crohn's disease.[216] It is startling that even with this early information, several attempts with plant-based, moderate to high carbohydrate diets were attempted to treat Crohn's disease.[217–219] Although each diet was met with modest success, the inflammatory condition remained and medical management was still required.

In a case study report in 2016 about a 14-year-old boy with severe Crohn's disease, the authors suggest the use of a paleolithic ketogenic diet.[220] Unlike the previous reports, this diet resulted in complete resolution of symptoms, normal blood labs, and gradual normalization of intestinal health. The teenager was able to discontinue all medication within two weeks and had remained on the diet for fifteen months without side effects at the time of the article. Without imaging, resolution of intestinal lymphatic inflammation cannot be known, but his results are suggestive that this was the case.

Celiac disease is a gastrointestinal disorder (also considered an autoimmune disorder) caused by a reaction to *gluten* (a group of various proteins found in wheat and in other grains such as barley and rye) that primarily affects the small intestine. An unusually strong immune response may lead to the production of several different antibodies leading to inflammation and the flattening of intestinal villi (tiny hair-like projections lining the inside of the small intestine which contain blood and lymph vessels). The damage to the villi affects the absorption of nutrients and can frequently lead to anemia and other deficiencies. Symptoms of celiac disease may include diarrhea, fatigue, weight loss, nausea, vomiting and abdominal bloating, gas and pain.

The lymphatic system is impacted in a variety of ways by celiac disease. Specialized lymphatic lacteals housed in the intestinal villi are responsible for the absorption of dietary fat. Depending on the severity of the condition, damage to these villi can impair the absorption of fat and fat-soluble vitamins and lead to deficiencies.[221] Due to the exaggerated immune response in celiac disease, lymphoid organs involved in immunity, such as the spleen, may be impacted. Several articles report shrinkage of the spleen, called splenic atrophy, associated with celiac disease.[222,223] Additionally, the excessive intestinal inflammation may encourage growth of new, possibly poorly developed, lymph vessels as seen with other chronic inflammatory conditions.

CROSS SECTION OF INTESTINAL CELL VILLI

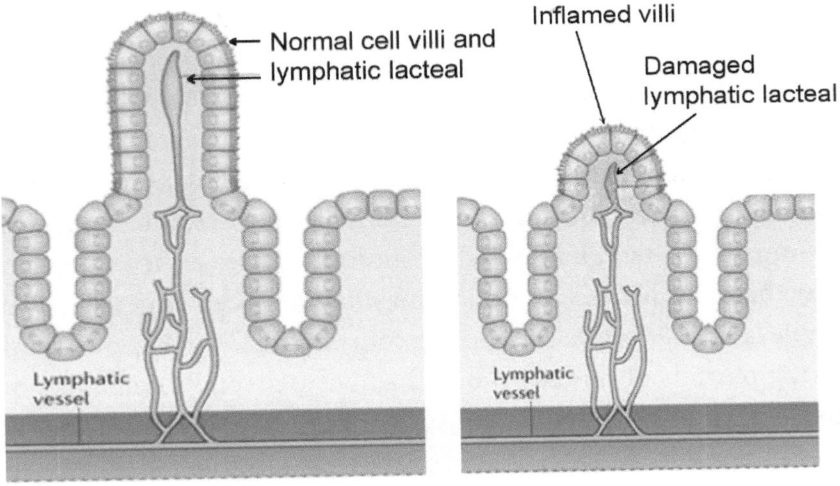

Figure 14. Normal and damaged intestinal villi and lacteals.

The majority of research and papers dealing with nutrition for celiac disease focus on a gluten-free diet[224,225] with surprisingly little study about how a ketogenic diet may affect this disorder. Grain of any kind is avoided in a well-formulated ketogenic diet and therefore can be a reasonable, and even optimal, choice for someone with celiac disease. Although a portion of people with celiac disease continue to have gastrointestinal symptoms,[226] complete avoidance of grains indefinitely may lead to intestine and lymphatic healing and resolution of celiac disease symptoms.

Autoimmune Diseases

Our immune system, of which our lymphatic system is a central participant, works to keep us safe from invaders like bacteria and viruses. When the immune system senses something foreign, it responds by sending out both generalized and highly specific fighter cells to neutralize the threat. Autoimmune disease is a condition in which the immune system mistakenly perceives normal healthy cells to be germs or toxins and attacks them. The symptoms of an autoimmune disease depend on which body system is being attacked. Discussed here will be rheumatoid arthritis, systemic lupus erythematosus (lupus), multiple sclerosis, and autoimmune thyroiditis (Hashimoto's disease).

In my own practice, it has not been unusual to observe patients with autoimmune diseases suffering from lower leg swelling. I had always assumed that this was an example of dependent edema due to immobility, as described in Chapter 3. With more research examining the impact of lymphatics in autoimmune disease, it is becoming clear that lymphatic dysfunction may have an even larger role than a simple lack of effective calf muscle contraction to aid lymph drainage during periods of illness-related inactivity. Several researchers have commented that the lymphatic system has a key role in autoimmune disease not only because it is primarily responsible for transporting immune cells to where they are needed, but also due to its role in evacuating harmful toxins from tissues.[227] A failure to do either job adequately can contribute to the development of an autoimmune disease.[228]

The role of lymphatics in **rheumatoid arthritis** is indicative of how dramatic the lymphatic-autoimmune disease connection is. The basis for lymphatic involvement in rheumatoid arthritis initially is due to inflammation, which stimulates the growth of new lymph vessels.[229] Unfortunately, the very toxic materials that are being removed by the lymphatic system in rheumatoid arthritis are damaging to the lymph vessels themselves and cause their collapse. This gradually results in a failure of the lymphatics to effectively remove toxic materials, leading to further inflammation and more joint damage.[230]

Because of its anti-inflammatory properties, a ketogenic diet has been suggested as a possible intervention for rheumatoid arthritis.[231]

Ketones, produced by the body either through fasting or carbohydrate restriction, have been shown to suppress inflammatory agents and reduce the symptoms of rheumatoid arthritis.[232,233]

Systemic lupus erythematosus, or lupus, is an autoimmune disease that attacks many different body systems and can have a wide range of presentations, making it especially difficult to diagnose. The most distinctive symptom found in many people with lupus is the facial rosacea (rash) that looks like butterfly wings across the center of the face. Although the connections between lymphatics and lupus are not very well studied, there are several case reports of patients with lupus who also suffer from lymphatic impairments such as *chylous ascites* (an accumulation of lipid-rich lymph in the abdominal cavity) and lymphedema.[229] Because of the inflammation associated with lupus, I believe the nature of lymphatic involvement in this condition will soon be better understood and articulated.

As with other autoimmune conditions, lupus may also respond well to eating a well-formulated ketogenic diet. In one six-week study, a comparison of a low glycemic diet versus a low-calorie, low-fat diet showed carbohydrate restriction to be beneficial for fatigue reduction and weight loss for participants diagnosed with lupus.[234] Additionally, the anti-inflammatory effects of the healthy fats consumed in a ketogenic diet would be beneficial for this condition.

Multiple sclerosis (MS) is a chronic and typically progressive condition involving damage to the *myelin sheath*, an insulating layer that allows electrical impulses to transmit quickly and efficiently along a nerve cell's tail-like extension or axon (see Figure 15 on next page). MS has been characterized as both an autoimmune disease in which the body's immune system attacks itself, and as a neurodegenerative disorder due to the gradual deterioration in the nervous system. People with multiple sclerosis may experience numbness, poor coordination, diminished vision, pain and fatigue. Particularly if confined to a wheelchair, people with multiple sclerosis may also experience lower body swelling. The severity of swelling may be related to the level of mobility restriction, with greater immobility also increasing the risk of blood clots.[235]

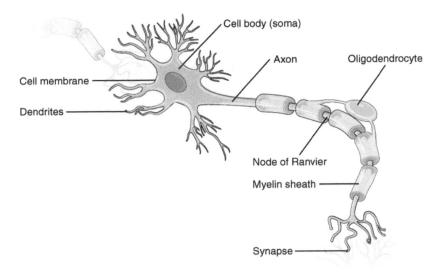

Figure 15. Nerve cell diagram showing axon and myelin sheath.

Storoni and Plant[236] theorize that lymphatic vessels are recruited in multiple sclerosis in response to chronic inflammation. They suggest that because of the myriad benefits with carbohydrate restriction and high healthy fat intake on mitochondrial function as well as its anti-inflammatory and neuroprotective properties, a ketogenic diet is an attractive option for people with multiple sclerosis. I would also suggest that another reason for the success of this dietary intervention is the healing effect of a ketogenic diet on lymphatic function.

Hashimoto's disease, or *autoimmune thyroiditis*, is characterized by an immune system attack on the thyroid gland. The thyroid gland is an endocrine organ responsible for coordinating many of the body's functions, including metabolism, growth, and development. Hashimoto's disease is a common cause of hypothyroidism, or low thyroid. Symptoms can include fatigue, cold sensitivity, weight gain, constipation, hair loss, dry skin, and depression.

There is some evidence of recruitment of new lymphatic vessels in response to inflammation as well as new lymph node-like structures in the neck that can be observed in Hashimoto's disease.[237] In a study of 199 patients with Hashimoto's disease, 184 had enlarged paratracheal lymph nodes while only 28 out of the 110 control subjects did.[238]

The thyroid gland drains to the paratracheal lymph nodes along the side of the neck. These nodes are part of the deep cervical nodes and can become swollen and sore during a cold or sore throat. Enlarged lymph nodes can suggest inflammation or an inflated immune response due to infection. The authors of this study suggested that ultrasound identification of enlarged paratracheal lymph nodes can be another method of diagnosing Hashimoto's disease.

Because the action of the thyroid gland is lowered upon rapid weight loss and this effect is known to be long-lasting,[239] thyroid function should be monitored when weight loss of more than ten percent of starting weight is a goal. A down-regulated thyroid results in a slower metabolism which will impede further weight loss attempts.[240] Even management of critical conditions like epilepsy using a ketogenic diet without any weight loss can result in lowered thyroid output.[241] It is unclear if the lower thyroid function is pathological or not. It may be that in the absence of symptoms, a blood panel test result outside of a normal reference range should not be the single determinant of the presence of thyroid disease.

It has been suggested that a reduction in thyroid hormone medication levels may be necessary when using a ketogenic eating plan. Although a ketogenic diet may be beneficial for lymphatic disorders, if low thyroid symptoms are present, medical management of hypothyroidism is recommended.

Obesity

The tremendous negative effect of obesity on the lymphatic system was the focus of my first book, *The Ketogenic Solution for Lymphatic Disorders:*

Lose Weight and Dramatically Reduce Lymphatic Swelling. Even as the obesity epidemic has become one of the world's greatest concerns, it has taken over the lymphatic and fat disorder community to an even greater degree. The Canadian data from the Lymphedema Impact and Prevalence International Study showed that 54.4 percent of participants had lymphedema due to obesity, second only to venous disease as a cause.[242] In Australia, the figure was 45 percent of participants.[243] The collective data from the United Kingdom, France, Italy, and Turkey showed 54 percent of participants were obese or morbidly obese.[244] The co-occurrence of lipedema and obesity is even higher at 85-88 percent in some papers.[73,79]

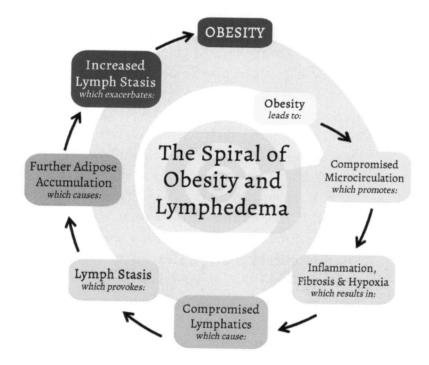

Figure 16. The spiral of obesity and lymphedema.

Obesity also increases the risk for many conditions besides lymphedema, including heart disease, diabetes, stroke, hypertension, sleep apnea, and some cancers. A massive meta-analysis of over ten million participants in 239 studies conducted between 1970 and 2015 in 32 countries found that for every five units of BMI increase above 25 kg/m², there was almost a 31 percent increased risk of premature death.[245] Even though participants were excluded from the study if they were a smoker or had any other comorbidities, participants still had a 49 percent higher risk for death from cardiovascular diseases, 38 percent from respiratory diseases, and 19 percent from cancer, if obesity was present.

Many experts have commented on the emerging data verifying the impact of obesity on lymphatic function and vice versa.[150,246] Figure 16 on the next page depicts the tragic spiral of obesity and lymphedema, with ever increasing weight leading to greater lymphatic failure while creating sometimes irreversible damage to body tissues and systems. It is also evident that lymphatic impairment can contribute to obesity by increasing the propensity for fat deposition.[246–248]

Clearly, a dietary option that is beneficial for both obesity and lymphatic disorders, such as a well-formulated ketogenic diet, is warranted. Recent compelling evidence regarding the idea that obesity impairs lymphatics but a high fat diet does not is being substantiated in research.[249,250] Thankfully, the era of dietary fat phobia is coming to an end. More research is being conducted regarding the efficacy of a ketogenic diet on a variety of conditions, including lymphatic and fat disorders.[251] Steve D. relates how his version of "hospital keto" reduced his weight and swelling:

> *"I was able to do what I call "hospital keto," which is the closest I could get to a true ketogenic diet, given my choices here. It worked! I lost 100 pounds in a year. Added to the 50 pounds I had managed to very slowly lose just by making wiser food choices, I'm down 150 pounds. My legs look normal for the first time in years. I still carry a lot of lymph fluid on the left side of my torso and my belly, but much less than before. I haven't had cellulitis again in ages and my skin is in much better condition." —Steve D.*

It is worth mentioning here that although many health conditions are associated with obesity, obesity is not their root cause. Insulin resistance, or a reduced response to the hormone insulin, is the fundamental reason for many chronic conditions,[252] and it has a negative influence on lymphatic health as well.[45] Scientist and pathophysiology professor Dr. Benjamin Bikman, in his bestselling book *Why We Get Sick*, explains how obesity is actually a downstream effect of insulin resistance. In the same way, cardiovascular disease, diabetes, neurodegenerative diseases and the other health issues discussed in this chapter are all symptoms of insulin resistance. By addressing the root of the problem, a well-formulated ketogenic diet may reverse disease and enhance lymphatic health.

To understand how a ketogenic diet can accomplish this, we must examine some nutrition basics. In the next chapter, we will take a look at the nutrient needs of the human body and how the lymphatic system is affected by various diets. Later, in Chapter 6, the basics of a ketogenic diet will be explained. These will be important pieces of the puzzle that we will use to further deduce the Lymphatic Code.

Chapter 5

Nutritional Evidence: Comparing Diets

"There is nothing like first-hand evidence."
Sir Arthur Conan Doyle, A Study in Scarlet

Because nutrition has such a significant effect on health, scientific studies of diet and nutrition are of supreme importance. Nutrition research is, however, notoriously difficult and challenging. Costs and personal human limitations often affect the study's duration and number of participants. Short studies with limited numbers of participants can't provide definitive results that support convincing conclusions. My own first foray into nutrition research suffered from this limitation. My sample size included only 12 participants and the intervention lasted just 3 months, so my conclusions could only suggest that a ketogenic diet for people with lymphatic disorders could be beneficial.[253]

But large, extended trials have challenges as well. Ensuring that a large group of people follows a specific dietary prescription over an extended time period is next to impossible. Many of the longer, broader (i.e., epidemiological) studies must rely upon the participants to fill out diet questionnaires, such as a dietary recall survey or food frequency questionnaire. These are notoriously inaccurate.[254] In one study, even receiving help from a trained professional did not substantially increase the accuracy of a 24-hour dietary recall.[255] Think about this for a second — what did you eat yesterday? Unless you wrote it down as you ate it, you most likely couldn't remember with complete accuracy. In fact, consider this most damning evidence of the unreliability of these surveys: an analysis of one of the most respected nutrition research projects, the National Health and Nutrition Examination Survey (NHANES), which has examined data from approximately 5,000 participants each year since 1999, revealed that two thirds of the data collected on energy intake (i.e, calories) from diet questionnaires was physiologically implausible and incompatible with life.[256,257]

Another limitation of dietary studies is in the management of confounding variables. One of the jobs of a research team is to control for variables which might affect their study's conclusions. For example, if a study seeks to examine the influence of protein intake on insulin levels, failure to control carbohydrate intake across participants would lead to inaccurate results because carbohydrates have such a dramatic impact on insulin.

One such uncontrolled study has had calamitous consequential repercussions on nutritional policy in the United States and eventually the rest of the world. Ancel Keys' now infamous Seven Countries study has propelled the "low-fat is good" dietary guidelines adopted by most countries around the world in the last four decades.[258] This study was riddled with variables unaccounted for during data collection. In particular, the conclusions of this study were based on food frequency questionnaires filled out by people not only recently ravaged by World War II, but also devoutly abstaining from meat consumption for an almost two-month long religious practice (Lent). Both of these highly significant confounding matters severely restricted the participants' food choices and caloric intake, which were then duly recorded on their surveys.[259]

Despite these limitations, it is still important to continue trying to educate ourselves about what may be the healthiest way to eat in general, as well as what may be optimal for each individual. My purpose here is also to discuss the potential impacts of an eating plan on the health of the lymphatic system.

Effect of Various Diets on the Lymphatics

Although I advocate for a particular way of eating in this book (a well-formulated ketogenic diet), I will offer the science of nutrition as it pertains to your lymphatic system by explaining what happens to the lymphatics when one follows different dietary regimes. With some understanding of the science of nutrition, you can choose which way of eating is healthier for you. Your dietary pattern may change over time with self-experimentation, continued learning, and, of course, depending on your circumstances. Although there are many other named diets, I've chosen the following seven as representative of recent popular ways of eating.

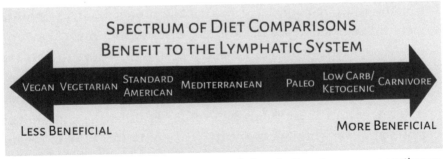

Figure 17: Ways of eating and their impact on the lymphatic system are on a continuum, and there is quite a bit of overlap among these different ways of eating. Generally, though, focusing on the right side of the list is more beneficial for lymphatics.

Vegan Diet

The Vegan Society website[260] defines veganism as a whole way of life, but in dietary terms, being a **vegan** means avoiding all foods that are "derived wholly or partly from animals." Because only plant-sourced foods are consumed, this diet is shown on Figure 17 at the farthest left position. Animal-derived foods, such as honey, eggs or dairy, are all excluded on a vegan diet. Manufactured plant foods such as industrialized seed oils (canola and corn oil) and "meat alternatives," that are loaded with additives, chemicals, and artificial sweeteners can be part of this eating plan. Many vegans, however, prefer instead to limit themselves to fresh, whole foods and may realize some health benefits, especially if their previous diet included common highly processed foods.

Even when a concerted effort is made to consume only organic, locally grown plants, long-term engagement in a vegan diet is likely the least healthy of the commonly promoted ways of eating. The possibility of multiple nutrient deficiencies exist, most notably vitamin B_{12}, which does not occur in plants at all. Other troubling deficiencies include: fat soluble vitamins (A, D, E, and K), creatine, carnitine, choline, and carnosine.[261,262]

Other nutrients are either not complete or are in a form that has a limited bioavailability to humans. Many plant sources of protein are too low in or missing one or more of the essential amino acids, and thus are considered incomplete protein sources. In order to avoid deficiencies, people who eat a vegan diet must develop a sophisticated knowledge and make a concerted effort to combine foods in specific ways so that all essential amino acids are consumed.

While some plant sources have complete proteins, such as soy and some grains, these foods have other health risks and are best consumed in very limited quantities, if at all.[128,263,264] Other notable examples of the poor bioavailability of nutrients in plants are omega-3 and omega-6 essential fatty acids. The forms of these nutrients found in plants are not accessible to human metabolic processes and must be converted in order to be used. This is an inefficient process in the human body, and may not always result in quantities sufficient for optimal health.[265] Similarly, while iron may be plentiful in some plants, its plant form (non-heme) is poorly absorbed, while heme iron, found only in animal-sourced foods, is highly available to humans and meets our needs in a superior fashion. Vegans have a higher risk of several conditions including leaky gut, anemia, depression, osteoporosis, nonalcoholic fatty liver disease, and eating disorders.[266-269]

The effect of a vegan diet on lymphatics is twofold. First, the lack of animal sourced foods limits access to complete proteins and bioavailable fats required for optimal lymphatic functioning. Second, a solely plant-based diet increases the volume of carbohydrates consumed, many of which are high in starches and sugars and are known to be inflammatory to lymphatics. As discussed previously, a consequence of inadequate protein consumption is hypoproteinemia, sometimes called edematous malnutrition (swelling due to malnutrition). Additionally, a common misconception is that because lymphedema is characterized by a high-protein edema, this necessitates eating a low-protein diet. But eating too little protein, or poor quality and incomplete proteins will actually exacerbate swelling.

Food items found on a vegan diet offer virtually nothing to support a robust lymphatic system. A vegan diet can only really be nutritious if one is educated enough to understand its deficiencies and rich enough to be able to afford costly supplements to replace those missing nutrients. As Dr. Benjamin Bikman, adipose tissue researcher at Brigham Young University says, a vegan diet is a "privilege of the elite." To be clear, the nutrient content in a vegan way of eating creates deficiencies that are difficult or impossible to correct.

Vegetarian Diet

The word "**vegetarian**" has come to be understood as someone who eats predominantly, but not exclusively, a diet of plant foods (shown on Figure 17 just to the right of a vegan diet). Most people who consider themselves vegetarian supplement their diets with some animal-sourced food, such as eggs, dairy, or even some fish or poultry. Vegetarianism seems to encompass an omnivorous diet of mostly plants with red meat the only thing really off the table. The newest term coined and used is "plant-based diet." This tends to be a more popular way of eating because it is both less restrictive and is often not connected to any strong moral beliefs as may be the case for adherents to veganism. There is, however, a very strongly held belief by those advocating for a vegetarian diet that consuming plants is healthier than eating animal-sourced foods. Yet, many of the health risks associated with a vegan diet are also a concern when using a vegetarian eating plan.[266-269]

The essential nutrients needed for a vigorous lymphatic system might be more readily obtained on a vegetarian rather than a vegan diet, but only through that portion that is animal-sourced. As I will discuss later in this chapter, a plant-based diet supplemented with eggs, fish, and some dairy, can also be ketogenic. In general though, a plant-based vegetarian diet tends to be too high in carbohydrates and is inflammatory to the lymphatic system. A healthy lymphatic system needs those essential nutrients that may be insufficient or entirely absent in a plant-based vegetarian diet.

Standard American Diet

The **Standard American Diet (SAD)** is the most common way of eating in the Western world and has been implicated in most, if not all, modern chronic diseases.[270] Plant-based foods are encouraged on the SAD, so this diet is still toward the left of center in Figure 17. This way of eating tends to be both high in carbohydrates and high in fats (despite recommendations of the Dietary Guidelines to eat very low fat), a particularly dangerous combination that can lead to metabolic syndrome and insulin resistance.[271] A corresponding rise in chronic conditions including diabetes, cardiovascular disease, obesity and cancer is associated with the adoption of the SAD, truly a horrendous nutritional catastrophe.

Although Americans were encouraged to eat a balanced diet from the Four Food Groups in 1956, more detailed information was provided when the Dietary Guidelines for Americans was first published in 1980, promoting widespread adoption of the SAD. The Guidelines are updated every five years, but very little has changed from the original version. Worse, any institution that receives federal funds must conform to the Dietary Guidelines. This includes the military, schools, prisons, hospitals and nutrition assistance programs through Social Services. All of these programs must comply with a Standard American Diet.

The Food Pyramid, first introduced in 1992, is the most familiar depiction of the Dietary Guidelines and the SAD. (MyPlate came out in 2011, but is essentially the same dietary plan). The base of the pyramid

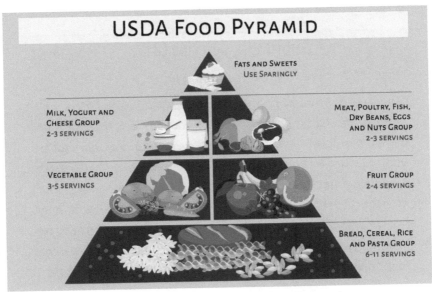

Figure 18. A representation of the USDA Food Pyramid (1992)

is grains and cereals with a recommendation that we consume 6-11 servings per day. Of note is that this group of foods has very little nutrition at all unless it is "fortified" with the vitamins and minerals it is lacking. The next level up is fruits and vegetables, a huge range of foods that include many that are very high in sugar and starch, with a recommendation of 6-8 total servings per day. If the plan is being followed, you may have already consumed 11 servings of bread, 5 carrots, and 4 apples before you get to anything of nutritional value in the pyramid.

The next level includes a low-fat dairy group and an equal sized group that includes meat, poultry, fish, beans, eggs and nuts. If you aren't already too full (or perhaps even if you are), you are instructed to have 2-3 servings of both of these groups. The top of the pyramid is reserved for eating "fats, oils & sweets...sparingly." The biggest portion of the pyramid on the lowest two levels is loaded with sugars and starches, so it's too late to comply with the limited sweets recommendation. And, equally disastrous for your lymphatic system, healthy fats and oils are severely restricted.

Calories In, Calories Out...

I recently received this disheartening note:

"There is one physical situation that is really annoying me. I can't get rid of my blubber. I exercise five or six days a week, I'm now using a rowing machine. I was using my bicycle on a stationary roller, but that wasn't working after two or three years, so I switched to the rowing machine. However I've been doing it for almost four months and still no change. I eat what I think is well, and only two meals a day. I think I'll switch to one meal a day and keep on rowing. That way my body will have to eat the blubber to get the fuel it needs for the exercise – at least I hope that's how it works."

This is an example of someone who believes in Calories In, Calories Out (CICO) as a strategy for losing weight. CICO is not an approach to losing weight, it is simply a description. Gary Taubes, the author of Good Calories, Bad Calories, explains this using an analogy of a bar with lots of people inside. To say that it is crowded because more people came in than went out is not addressing the reasons why the bar is crowded. Maybe the movie next to the bar just let out. Maybe people were enticed to enter because it was happy hour. Establishing the cause is key to developing an effective and healthy true weight loss strategy.

Mediterranean Diet

Similar to the SAD is the "**Mediterranean diet.**" This is a poorly defined, nebulous concept that seems to suggest that the entire Mediterranean region has a common way of eating. The Mediterranean spans from Slovenia in the north, Israel and Egypt to the east, Libya to the south, and Morocco and Spain to the west. Though all of these countries border the Mediterranean, they have vastly differing climates and cultures as well as widely divergent ways of eating. In Egypt for instance, their diet is heavily based on cereals, while in Spain there is little grain and quite a lot of meat and seafood.

A review seeking to define what constitutes a Mediterranean diet noted the incredible variations found in studies that sought to attribute health benefits to the diet.[272] The authors found that the quantity of servings in each food category could range from one to thirteen and adherence to the diet could be rated anywhere from 22 percent to 87 percent depending on diet definition and scoring methods. In their conclusion, the authors maintain that "high level evidence" exists for the effectiveness of the Mediterranean Diet to "improve cardiovascular and cognitive health," yet this seems impossible without any actual agreed upon description of the diet.

Figure 19 on the next page suggests one commonly advanced definition. Not only does this figure give very little specific direction, it is alarmingly carbohydrate and plant heavy. Except for severe limitations on red meat consumption, this Mediterranean diet description seems to have very little difference from the food choices recommended in the USDA food pyramid and the SAD and so it is placed closely with the SAD in Figure 17. The guidance to consume more sweets than red meat is astonishing. Red meat is limited to 4 servings a month while it is recommended that sweets should be consumed 3 servings per week! In studies comparing health benefits, a so-called Mediterranean diet had modest improvements compared to those of the SAD.[273,274] And despite the lack of specificity in a Mediterranean diet, studies comparing the outcomes of this vague way of eating to outcomes of a ketogenic diet showed significantly better results in the ketogenic diet groups.[275,276]

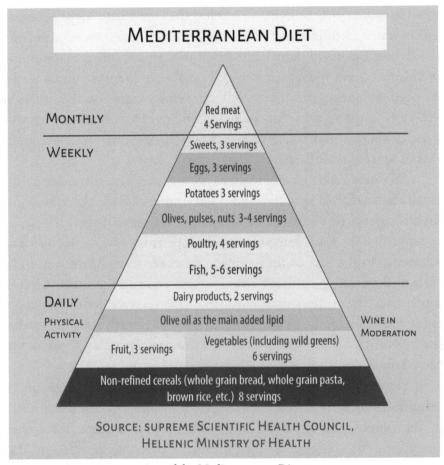

Figure 19. One representation of the Mediterranean Diet

As with the several diets already discussed, I believe the Mediterranean diet may still have deleterious effects on the lymphatic system. This is primarily due to its restriction on the consumption of saturated fat, red meat and other animal-sourced foods and its promotion of high levels of carbohydrate intake, including the encouragement of harmful grains and starchy vegetables.

Paleo Diet

The **Paleo Diet** was developed in the latter part of the last century from research into the archeological record and study of modern hunter-gatherer populations. Proponents of a Paleo diet assert that a return to how humans ate prior to the adoption of agriculture may be a healthier diet than current practices.[277] Walter Voegtlin was the first to publish a book about paleolithic nutrition called *The Stone Age Diet* (1975). Later, S. Boyd Eaton is credited as one of the originators of the Paleo diet due to his article published in the respected *The New England Journal of Medicine* in 1985 that explored the nutritional evolution of humans in search of how and what we are meant to eat.[278] The "modern" Paleo diet gained more traction with best selling books by Dr. Loren Cordain, an exercise physiologist, and Robb Wolf, an exercise and nutrition researcher, as well as the promotion of this diet by many Crossfit trainers. Although the CrossFit organization does not currently support a single diet, for some time the two were closely associated.[279]

Despite evidence that shows that the diet of early humans was dependent upon local resources (tropical populations ate more fruit, people living near water consumed more marine life, and northernmost groups ate almost exclusively animal-sourced foods for much of the year), the Paleo diet strives to make a general prescription for modern populations. Also troubling is the fact that modern day versions of both plants and animals are quite different from those of prehistoric, or even of relatively more recent Medieval periods. Modern day plants have been hybridized for a greater sugar or starch content,[280] (see Figure 20 on next page) while domesticated animals are much fattier than the wild animals hunted by our ancestors. The effort is commendable but may not give enough sound direction to allow for optimal nutrition and health.

Recommendations for this diet include: lean meats, vegetables, fruits, and honey. Excluded are all grains, dairy products, processed foods, added sugar and sugar substitutes, and alcohol. This puts the paleo diet in the middle of the diet continuum, but only because it advocates for whole foods and eliminates all grains – much better recommendations than the diets farther to the left. The inclusion of high glycemic fruits, starchy vegetables and honey, though, may prove to be too inflammatory for the lymphatic system. The across-the-board elimination of all dairy, an excellent source of healthy dietary fat that may be essential for lymphatics, is equally unfortunate.

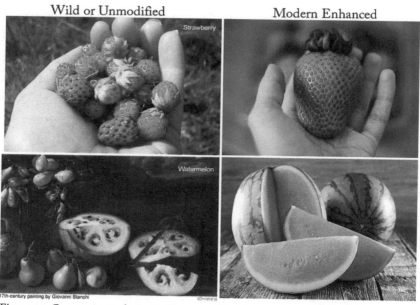

Figure 20. Comparison of genetically unmodified fruit to modern enhanced versions. Watermelons are from oil paintings by Giovanni Stanchi Dei Fiori circa 1645-1672 (from Giovanni Stanchi Wikimedia Commons).

Low Carbohydrate Diet and the Ketogenic Lifestyle

Over the past couple of hundred years, the idea of eating a **low carbohydrate diet** has been discussed and used to treat various diseases including type 1 diabetes, epilepsy, and obesity.[281,282] The concept of using carbohydrate restriction for weight loss has been known at least as far back as William Banting's *Letter on Corpulence* from 1869. This rotund undertaker asked his doctor what he could do to feel better and lower his weight. His doctor suggested that he cut out carbohydrates. Banting took the wise advice to heart and, when he experienced superb results with weight loss and the easing of his other ailments, he wrote what may be the very first diet book.[283]

In recent years, since Dr. Robert Atkins popularized the clinical use of a low carbohydrate diet, the benefit of carbohydrate restriction has become more widely known. The acceptance of a low carbohydrate diet is bringing health and vitality to a whole new generation.

A **ketogenic diet** is called such because of its effect in generating *ketones*, fatty acid metabolites that can be used as an efficient energy source. When your body switches from burning sugar to burning fat (either stored body fat or dietary fat) as its main fuel source, you are in *ketosis*. Fat-burning, or ketosis, is halted in the presence of insulin. Remember that insulin levels are higher when carbohydrates are consumed, but with severe carbohydrate restriction, insulin levels drop and ketosis can occur. Ketosis is certainly effective for losing weight (even for conditions like lipedema which was previously thought to be impervious to diet) but, as previously discussed in this book, research has shown that the power of ketone molecules themselves is extensive for restoring and maintaining health in general and in particular for the lymphatic system.

A low-carbohydrate diet is not necessarily ketogenic, so it is important to compare and contrast the two diets. The main difference between the two is the amount of carbohydrates allowed. A low-carb diet consists of 10-35 percent of calories in carbohydrate, or about 50 to 150 grams of carbohydrates per day, while a ketogenic diet allows no more than 20 grams of carbohydrate per day. Since the typical Western diet can include as much as 65 percent of calories from carbohydrates, or 325 grams per day, a decrease to even 150 grams is still a substantial decrease and may lead to great health benefits.[284] Both low-carb and ketogenic diets eliminate grains, starchy vegetables and sugary beverages, and both encourage increased consumption of healthy fats as an energy source.

Because plant-based foods are higher in carbohydrate than animal-sourced foods, it is easier for a vegan or vegetarian to conform to a low carb diet rather than a ketogenic eating plan. In my opinion, it is virtually impossible to follow both a vegan diet and a well-formulated ketogenic diet because of the tremendous challenge of keeping carbohydrates low enough while still consuming enough protein.

Low-carbohydrate and ketogenic diets are on the right hand, or preferable, end of the diet continuum shown in Figure 17. Limitation in carbohydrate intake along with consumption of adequate complete proteins from animal sources and plenty of healthy fat makes these eating plans exceptionally health-promoting. Traci J. notes the many benefits she realized when she changed to a ketogenic eating plan with the guidance of her new doctor:

"I was referred to a great doctor here in Arizona who has actually written a book on a keto way of eating and since my first visit…[I] have lost 32 pounds! … I just feel so much better overall…My thyroid levels, estrogen, and progesterone levels were all out of whack! But now, my levels are so much better. My progesterone level was so low, it wasn't detected. I'm sleeping better, no more hot flashes! I have energy to do lymphatic yoga in the morning, jump on my rebounder for 10 minutes and get on my vibration plate for 15 minutes, all before going to work!…Now I don't have swelling in my legs and feet and no more shooting pain in my thigh…" —Traci J.

Carnivore Diet

The **carnivore diet** is on the opposite end of the spectrum from a vegan diet, as this way of eating includes only animal-sourced foods. This may include any kind of meat (beef, pork, lamb etc), poultry, fish and shellfish, dairy products, and eggs. Some strict adherents eat only beef, salt, and water and claim this to be the "perfect elimination diet." The extreme limitation in food variety and the practice of introducing new foods one at a time makes it much easier to determine food intolerances.

There has been very little study on the carnivore way of eating although a great deal of documentation exists of healthy northern populations subsisting on a predominantly meat-based or animal-sourced diet for most of the year.[285] Perhaps the most detailed study regarding a carnivore diet was performed in 1928-1929 on two Arctic explorers, Vilhjalmur Stefansson and Karsten Andersen. After spending years "living off the land" with Inuit groups during extreme northern explorations, they agreed to participate in an all-meat diet while sequestered in the metabolic ward at Bellevue Hospital in New York.[286] The year-long study allowed the men to sleep at home but take all meals at the hospital except for two extended periods of time when they remained in the hospital overnight for several weeks. An incredible amount of data was collected and the results seemed to indicate that, at least for these two men, the diet did not result in any nutrient deficiencies or organ dysfunction. In fact, they finished the experiment healthier than when they started. Gingivitis resolved for Stefansson, and Andersen's blood pressure improved. Stefansson describes his "Adventures in Diet" in an article of that name which appeared in *Harper's Monthly Magazine* in 1935. A link is provided in the Resources section of this book.

What Stefansson and Andersen learned from living with the Inuit for many years was that all the nutrients a human needs can be obtained from meat and the fat that naturally comes with it.[285] Even vitamin C, previously believed to only come from fruits and vegetables, is provided for in this diet. For links to more detailed information about how all essential vitamins and minerals are met on a carnivore diet, please see the Resources section of this book.

Anecdotally, a carnivore diet has been found to be beneficial for several health conditions including gastrointestinal disorders, autoimmune diseases, metabolic disorders, mental illness and more. Because the carnivore diet is ultra low in carbohydrates (less than five grams per day), many women with lipedema experiment with carnivore when they find that a ketogenic diet is not low enough in carbohydrates to allow them to burn fat on the lower body.

Additionally, all plants have anti-nutrients and other toxins that are tolerated in varying levels by each individual. A diet that excludes all plants can effectively eliminate the introduction of any plant toxins, no matter how well tolerated. Lastly, hunger and cravings are completely managed by the satiation created by protein and fat. The improved response to satiety signals to the brain helps curb appetite and may be beneficial for managing eating disorders.

Finding the Ideal Diet: The Case For Animal-Sourced Food

The elements of an ideal diet, according to Dr. Paul Saladino in his book *The Carnivore Code*, must include all nutrients humans need to function optimally, in the most bioavailable form, with the smallest amount of toxins, while also keeping insulin low for long periods. It may be that these conditions can be met best when eating predominantly, or even exclusively, foods derived from animals.

Although a range of plant to animal-sourced eating plans can be considered ketogenic, in general eating more foods derived from animals will have more health benefits and may improve lymphatic functioning as well. The growing population of those experimenting and sustaining a carnivore diet teaches us that its benefits can be attributed to both eating more meat and also from consuming fewer plants.[285] The concept of gaining health from a plant-free diet may be difficult to accept initially, as it is in complete opposition to what most people have held to be true for the last 100 years.

Long standing platitudes you can't live by include: *eat a balanced diet, eat the rainbow,* and *eating fat makes you fat.* What do these statements mean and where did they come from? Until the Northern Inuits were exposed to Western culture, these people subsisted almost exclusively on hunted meats for most of the year. Some Pacific Islander populations ate only breadfruit, coconut, and fish. Clearly these diets were not balanced, colorful, nor do they have much variety in the modern sense, yet these people have thrived. We have also been admonished to eat in moderation. This nebulous rule produces circular thinking. The individual who becomes obese must not have eaten in moderation — because they are fat. All of these vague and unhelpful platitudes for eating are virtually impossible to follow because the concepts of "balance" and "moderation" are not measurable.

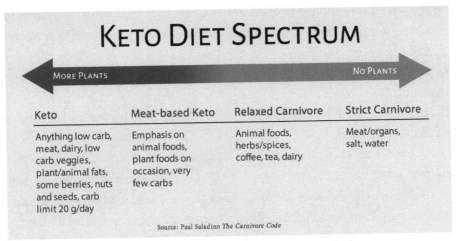

Figure 21. A range of plant-based to animal-sourced ketogenic foods.

In reality, these eating decrees only came into being after the advent of large agribusiness brought about the ability to purchase any plant food, during any season, from any location. As plant foods began to dominate our diet, careful planning was required to balance or pair certain foods together to ensure requirements for essential nutrients were met. Staple foods of the Western diet, such as bread, contain little or no nutrient value and have to be fortified with vitamins to avoid population-wide nutrient deficiencies. Regrettably, the practices of balance, moderation and variety, being impossible to follow, are never quite accomplished and have allowed many modern chronic diseases to flourish. I believe that just because we are able to gain some essential nutrients from plant sources doesn't mean we should do so. Amber O'Hearn, a data scientist and author who has been eating a plant-free diet for over a decade, states, *"Although we can make use of plants as a nutrient source, we don't have to, and in some cases we are better off minimising plant intake".[285]*

Biochemistry vs. Bio-Individuality.

There are two similar sounding concepts that are commonly mistaken for each other: biochemistry and bio-individuality. On occasion, a client will tell me, "My body doesn't work like that." But in actuality our biochemistry, the chemical and physiological processes that occur in a living being, is much more similar than it is different from person to person. Healthy human metabolism, that is, how the body takes in the chemicals from food and either burns them, or builds parts with them, or stores them for later, is relatively the same for all members of the human race.

Looking at a basic level, our cells need certain chemicals or nutrients in order to function. If the proper substances are not available in the correct form or in adequate amounts, cells are not able to function optimally. This is a common characteristic of all cells in the body. It is true, however, that if one preferred substance is not available, our clever bodies can, in certain circumstances, substitute a different chemical for that missing chemical, but the cell or organ will run the risk over time of becoming compromised. Substitution should only be a stopgap measure until the body receives what it actually needs. An example of this phenomenon is in the body's cell walls. The preferred substance for cell wall construction is cholesterol.[287] If adequate cholesterol is not available, the body will incorporate other fats in its place. This can work in the short term but the strength of those cell walls will be compromised and over time will function poorly and break down more easily. This is biochemistry and it applies to all humans.

A completely different concept from biochemistry is bio-individuality. Two individuals could consume all they need to function optimally, and yet be eating completely different things. One person might love spinach, eggs and fish, while another enjoys cauliflower, cheese and beef. Both people are eating an optimal diet, but may never eat identical foods. Bio-individuality accounts for preferences, intolerances, and allergies that may come about due to cultural, genetic, social, environmental, and geographical influences. These are the things which make us unique beings and we should celebrate them.

A major factor in bio-individuality is *immune tolerance*. Humans exhibit variation in how much of assorted toxins can be tolerated by their immune system. Urushiol, for instance, is the toxic chemical in poison oak that can cause an immune system reaction ranging from a very mild rash to oozing blisters. The degree of reaction depends on individual levels of immune tolerance. Similarly, the immune reaction demonstrated in lactose intolerance, gluten sensitivity, or a peanut allergy can range from little or no response at all to anaphylactic shock.[288] Your lymphatic system is a vital part of the immune system and can become overwhelmed by repeated exposure to toxins, resulting in inflammation and swelling. Therefore, avoiding foods that you have a sensitivity to is important to the health of your lymphatic system and to your general health.

Nutrient Density and Bioavailability.

Foods from animal sources would be exceptionally nutrient dense, if this term could be defined by a ratio of the amount of available nutrients to the size of the package. Beef liver, for instance, has 3.5 milligrams of iron in a small 3-ounce serving (about ¼ cup). Comparatively, five cups of spinach would need to be consumed to get the same amount of iron. The accepted definition of nutrient density is, however, *a ratio of nutrient amount to total calories in a serving of a particular food.* This is a less useful definition because it doesn't take into account the bioavailability of the nutrients. The non-heme iron present in spinach is not easily absorbed and so most of this nutrient is not available to be used by the body. Contrast this with the fact that all of the heme iron in beef liver is in the proper form and can easily be absorbed. Nutrient density without consideration for the bioavailability of that nutrient to humans is simply not meaningful.[289]

Essential Nutrients.

Wherever you decide to be on the spectrum of carbohydrate and plant intake, there can be no mistaking the fact that every human being requires certain nutrients that must be consumed. Essential nutrients are those that are required for life but either can't be produced by the body at all or not in adequate amounts. There are essential nutrients of three different types: Fatty acids (fats), amino acids (proteins), and micronutrients (vitamins and minerals). Remember, one of the requirements of an ideal diet is that it provides all nutrients humans need to function optimally. All essential nutrients are provided in a bioavailable form in foods derived from animals and, more importantly, some essential nutrients can only be found in animal sources. There are no essential nutrients that are exclusively found in plants.

Vitamin B_{12} is only found in animal-sourced foods in amounts adequate for humans. Although nori seaweed provides some bioavailable B_{12}, it is inadequate on its own, so vegans will need supplementation to avoid a deficiency.[290] The skin produces vitamin D from sunlight but if sun exposure is limited, it means that food and supplements must make up the shortfall. The form of vitamin D (D_3 - cholecalciferol) most beneficial to humans is only found in animal and fungal food sources. D_2 is found in fortified foods, such as bread, and is less efficiently utilized by cells.[291] Because food sources have limited vitamin D in general, supplementation is recommended, especially if animal-sourced foods are not consumed. Although considered non-essential because the body can produce small amounts, nutrients such as creatinine, carnosine, and taurine are only found exclusively in food derived from animals. These nutrients are vital for brain and muscle function and are usually deficient in those who consume only plant products.[292–294]

Docosahexaenoic acid (DHA) is an essential omega-3 fatty acid that is almost exclusively found in fish. Limited amounts can be found in a certain microalgae that can then be made into a supplement for vegans.[295] Another strategy employed by vegans is to use the plant-sourced omega-3 fatty acid alpha-linolenic acid (ALA) and rely on its conversion to DHA in the body. This is a very inefficient process, however, leaving most vegans with a DHA deficiency unless supplementation is used.[296,297]

Consuming a predominantly plant-based diet may pose an additional challenge. The lymphatic system is responsible for transport of fat-soluble vitamins which need the intake of fat in order for satisfactory amounts to be absorbed. The limited fat intake recommended in most plant-based dietary guidelines may result in deficiencies of the fat-soluble vitamins A, D, E and K.[298,299] An animal-sourced diet encourages eating the fat that comes naturally with animal products and has ample levels of the essential fat-soluble vitamins.

Plant Toxins and Anti-Nutrients

Lacking the ability to run away from predators, plants have developed unique methods of protecting themselves. One such protection is the use of plant toxins. Interestingly, 99 percent of toxins in the plant foods we consume are inherent in the plant themselves and not from pesticides or herbicides that may have been used during their production.[300] A plant can mount a chemical defense that may first appear as a bitter taste that deters an animal from eating it. If, however, the plant is still consumed despite an unpleasant taste, the dose and concentration of toxins increase, leading to various degrees of mild gastrointestinal distress, to paralysis or to death.[301] Table 1 lists the most common plant toxins, the plants they are found in, and symptoms associated with toxicity.

Plant Toxin	Common Foods	Symptoms of Toxicity
Alkaloids (nightshades)	tomatoes, peppers, eggplant	itching, nausea, vomiting, mild gastrointestinal perturbation, psychosis, paralysis, teratogenicity, arrhythmias and sudden death

Lectins	legumes, squash, nightshades	skin rashes, joint pain, general inflammation, flatulence, nausea, diarrhea, and vomiting
Cyanogenic Glycosides	tapioca root, flax, lima beans	headache, tightness in throat and chest, muscle weakness and death
Terpenoids	citrus, pepper, lemon grass	hematuria, renal failure, loss of vision, chest pain, vomiting, severe coughing, gastroesophageal hemorrhage, hypotension, swelling of the throat and even death[302]
Phenolics (tannins, flavanols)	chocolate, tea, berries, avocado, wine	stomach irritation, nausea, and vomiting; fever, anemia from breakdown of red blood cells, and hives
Salicylates	almonds, berries, coffee, cucumbers, pickles	nausea, vomiting, diaphoresis, tinnitus, vertigo, hyperventilation, tachycardia, and hyperactivity; as toxicity progresses, agitation, delirium, hallucinations, convulsions, lethargy, and stupor may occur
Phytates	most nuts and all types of beans	impairs the absorption of iron, zinc and calcium and may promote mineral deficiencies
Protease Inhibitors	cabbage, cucumbers, spinach, tomatoes	changes in how foods taste, fat redistribution, diarrhea, insulin resistance, high blood sugar, cholesterol and/or triglyceride levels, liver problems, nausea
Oxalates	spinach, almonds, cashews, cocoa powder	joint pain, muscle aches, fatigue, strange rashes, kidney stones, chronic UTIs, interstitial cystitis or kidney infections, cloudy or hazy urine, vulvar pain in women

Table 1. Common Plant Toxins

With proper preparation, the toxicity of some plants can be reduced, but might not be completely eliminated. For instance, soaking beans overnight and then cooking them reduces the impact of the toxin lectin found in them, but many people will still suffer from gas and flatulence after eating them.

Anti-nutrients are a category of plant toxins that interfere with the absorption of other essential nutrients. These plant compounds, found especially in grains, beans, legumes and nuts, can interfere with adequate absorption of essential vitamins and minerals such as zinc, iron, magnesium and calcium.[303] Similarly, protease inhibitors can diminish protein digestion, and the glucose molecule found in all carbohydrates, diminishes vitamin C absorption. Because vitamin C is vital for wound healing and immune functions, the lymphatic system may be further stressed when lacking the support of adequate vitamin C levels, leaving the individual immunocompromised.

Well-known for their role as the most common cause of kidney stones, the needle-shaped spiked structures of plant oxalates damage cells with which they come into contact. Plant foods such as spinach, almonds, kale, carrots, beans, beets, and many others are quite high in oxalates, yet animal foods contain little if any. If you are prone to kidney stone formation, it is good practice to avoid eating plants that have a high oxalate content.

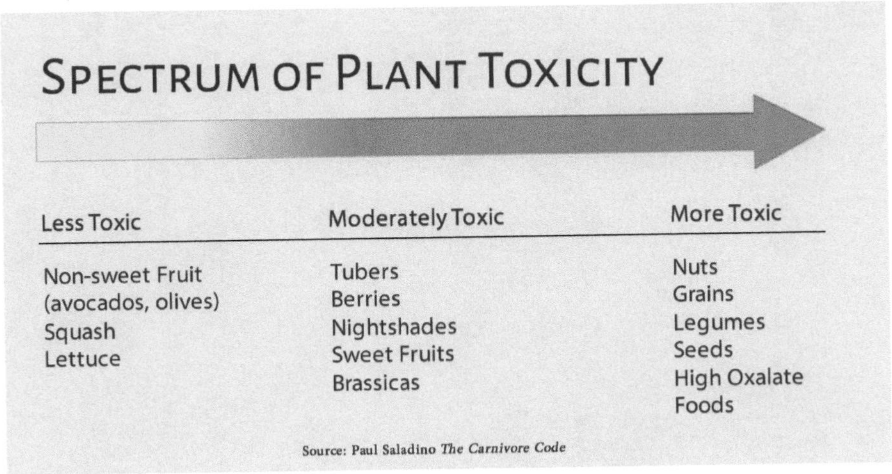

SPECTRUM OF PLANT TOXICITY

Less Toxic	Moderately Toxic	More Toxic
Non-sweet Fruit (avocados, olives)	Tubers	Nuts
Squash	Berries	Grains
Lettuce	Nightshades	Legumes
	Sweet Fruits	Seeds
	Brassicas	High Oxalate Foods

Source: Paul Saladino *The Carnivore Code*

Figure 22. The spectrum of plant toxicity

There are many issues to consider when eating to support a healthy lymphatic system. From what I've presented to this point, Sherlock Holmes would deduce that the most important consideration is keeping his carbohydrate consumption low and getting plenty of healthy fat along with adequate complete protein. That will inevitably lead him to ketogenic nutrition. In the next chapter, we'll see what Mr. Holmes needs to know to put this into practice.

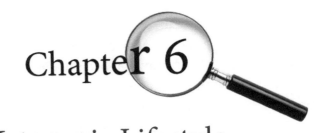

Chapter 6

Ketogenic Lifestyle Explained

"By George!" cried the inspector. "How did you ever see that?"
"Because I looked for it."
—Sir Arthur Conan Doyle, *The Adventure of the Dancing Men*

Before the advent of agriculture and the push to avoid animal sources of food in favor of a less natural plant-based diet, healthy eating used to come instinctually. We didn't need to research and study nutrition, we just ate. The further we became removed from the sources of our food by hunting and gathering in a grocery store instead of on the tundra or plains, the less we understood about which foods would make our lives better. Like Mr. Holmes, now we have to look for it in order to see it. In this chapter, I will give you the basics of ketogenic nutrition that will hopefully allow you to feed your lymphatics and lead a healthier life.

Tasks of the Three Macronutrients

As discussed in Chapter 5, one of the reasons that it's important to pay attention to what we eat is because there are specific nutrients necessary to life that our bodies can't produce. These are called essential nutrients. The following discussion will focus on the functions of protein, fat and carbohydrate, and I'll include some information about the essential nutrients within those macronutrient categories.

Protein

Protein, made up of essential and non-essential amino acids, is primarily used for building body tissues such as bones, muscles and cell walls, along with forming the basis for enzymes, antibodies, and hormones. Protein can be used for energy, but that is not its primary function and so it is the last macronutrient to be used as a fuel source. When necessary, protein can be converted by an inefficient process called gluconeogenesis into a form that the body can then burn and use for energy.

Is it imperative that humans consume protein? Emphatically yes. The body is continually breaking down and reusing proteins from various tissues. During the course of this action, a certain amount of protein is broken down and discarded in the urine. But in order to maintain health and function, your body constantly makes new combinations of proteins, most of which are made from proteins that were previously used for another purpose within your body. However, at least one third of protein structures within the body are produced from essential amino acids in the diet. If one's diet doesn't include adequate amounts of complete protein, eventually the protein necessary and available to rebuild the body will be insufficient, resulting in major health consequences.[285] One condition, as discussed in Chapter 3, is low protein levels in the blood (hypoproteinemia) which results in increased lymphatic load and swelling in the lower body. Other health effects of a low protein intake may include fatty liver disease, osteoporosis, kidney failure, muscle atrophy, and compromised immune function. In one study, participants with kidney disease consuming a very low protein diet had an increased risk of death.[304]

Consuming a high protein diet has health effects as well, such as a reduction in hunger, body weight, and percent body fat, each of which are regarded as advantageous.[305-307] What is considered high protein? The Recommended Daily Allowance (RDA) of protein suggested by the Food and Nutrition Board of the National Academy of Science is 0.8

grams per kilogram of body weight. But this amount can be increased to at least double (1.6 grams/kg), and perhaps higher, without risk of unfavorable responses in healthy individuals with normal kidney function.[308] Additionally, there is evidence to show that higher levels of protein intake may have beneficial effects for healing from trauma or surgery or to break a weight loss stall.[309]

Fat

Dietary fat, composed of essential and non-essential fatty acids, is an important fuel source for the body. Essential fatty acids are involved in many physiological processes such as blood clotting, wound healing, inflammation, and regulation of immune function and blood pressure. Fats are also used as a component of cell walls, keeping the cells supple. Fat is a carrier for the fat-soluble vitamins A, D, E and K, and supports their absorption into the body. Additionally, fat is used in the body as the basis of many hormones. Essential fatty acids are vital for proper neurological and vision development in infants, and for the maintenance of cognition and memory in adults. Dietary fat stimulates the lymphatic system and increases transport capacity by accelerating lymph flow.[94,99]

Fat's main job, however, is as a clean burning energy source, and it is the most efficient fuel of the three macronutrients at this job. With more than twice the energy per weight as either protein or carbohydrate, fat is also the cleanest fuel source for the body, creating the fewest toxins during its combustion.[310]

Dietary fat has several qualities that make it ideal for cooking as well as an enhancement for food appearance, taste, and texture. When foods are coated with fats, they have an appealing glossy and moist appearance. The moistness of fat also gives a pleasant lubricating mouthfeel that facilitates swallowing. Flavors that are only carried in fat alter the taste to something that is unique. For instance, if lamb and beef are stripped of all of their fat, the two meats are indistinguishable. Fats have important roles in making food satisfying and delaying the feeling of hunger for a longer time than would either protein or carbohydrate.

A deficiency in essential fatty acids can lead to a scaly rash, increased susceptibility to infection, poor wound healing, vision problems and neurological conditions such as neuropathy. Infants who are fed formula with inadequate essential fatty acids are at risk for poor brain development and visual disability.[311]

Other signs of a fatty acid deficiency include dry eyes, feeling constantly cold, dry hair and/or hair loss, hormonal problems including loss of menstrual cycle, difficulty concentrating, fat-soluble vitamin deficiency, and constant fatigue. Conversely, adequate intake of healthy dietary fat leads to increased levels of energy and a feeling of vitality, healthy hair, skin and nails, improved brain function, and reduced hunger.

Fats can be classified by how saturated their molecules are. A saturated fat has all of its carbon bonds taken up (saturated) with hydrogen, preventing oxygen from attaching itself (called oxidation). Oxidation is essentially the process of rusting or becoming rancid. This means that saturated fats are the most stable and the least likely to go bad. This is why your grandmother was able to leave cooking lard on the counter. It would not go bad even without refrigeration. Animal sources of fat are made up largely of saturated fat and are typically solid at room temperature. The most common plant source of saturated fat is coconut. Monounsaturated fat is less stable, but still only has one double bond for oxygen to attach to, making this also a healthy fat found in most animal sources. Other examples of monounsaturated fats are olive and avocado oil. Polyunsaturated fats (having many double bonds) are the least stable and care is required to keep them from becoming tainted. Healthy examples of polyunsaturated fats are those high in omega-3 fatty acids, such as fish oils. Other polyunsaturated fats include omega-6 varieties which are healthy in smaller amounts. The unhealthful varieties are heat-treated and chemically-processed oils such as corn, canola, and soybean oils. Omega-6 oils are known to be highly inflammatory[312,313] and may be especially so for the lymphatic system.

Fats can also be classified by how long of a molecule they are, such as short, medium, or long chain. The vast majority of the fats we consume are long chain fats including animal and fruit fats as well as omega-6 and omega-3 polyunsaturated fats. In the body, these fats are packaged into chylomicrons and transported by the lymphatic system to the blood. Medium chain fats are discussed most often in the context of lymphatics. Unlike long chain triglycerides, these fats bypass the intestinal lymphatics (lacteals) and are instead transported directly to the liver for fast energy via the portal vein. The most common foods high in medium chain fats include coconut and palm oil as well as grass-fed butter and other dairy.

Short chain fats are largely a product of fermentation of fiber by our gut bacteria. We don't eat short chain fats directly, except in the case of vinegar, which is made up of a short chain fat called acetic acid. Perhaps because of the ability of vinegar to stimulate the production of mitochondria (the powerhouse of the cell) and to improve glucose regulation and insulin sensitivity, this is why pickle juice is claimed to help with sugar cravings.

Carbohydrate

The third macronutrient is **carbohydrate**. Its job in the body is almost exclusively to be burned for energy. It does not play a significant role in building any physical components of the body. Carbohydrates are simply burned for energy. That's it. Because the body can produce the small amount of glucose it needs for the few types of cells that can't use protein or fat for fuel, there really is no biological need for consuming carbohydrates. This means there are no essential carbohydrates. As Dr. Robert Cywes, known as the Carb Addiction Doc, says, "Nobody dies if they don't eat carbohydrates".[314]

Essentially, the whole concept of calories was invented to help control the portion size when eating carbohydrates. In the 1820s, scientist Nicolas Clément was tinkering around in his lab, as they did during the golden age of basic scientific research, and developed several innovations in chemistry. One was his invention of the bomb calorimeter, used to measure the amount of heat generated from burning various substances such as wood or volatile chemicals. Over time, Clément tested several types of foods and an interesting trend was revealed. When he incinerated carbohydrates, they gave off a certain amount of heat. When he incinerated proteins, they gave off the same amount of heat per weight as did carbohydrates. But when he incinerated fat, it gave off two and a quarter times more heat as the same amount of either carbohydrates or protein. This is why your nutrition calculator tells you that a gram of carbohydrates has four calories while a gram of lard has nine. Does this mean that when lard is eaten, the body will gain two and a quarter times more weight than when an equal amount of starchy potato or lean meat is consumed? No. The first thing to keep in mind is that the human body is not a bomb calorimeter. It is a chemical factory and the action of food in the body is more than just creating heat and energy. Additionally, proteins, fats, and carbohydrates all behave differently in the body, with carbohydrates stimulating fat storage, while fat and protein stimulate fat burning. This will be discussed in more detail next.

The ability to calculate calories of various foods gave rise to the idea that eating fewer calories, or less food, would prevent obesity. But calorie counting is only useful in a diet high in carbohydrate because, unlike protein and fat, carbohydrate intake has no feedback mechanism to signal that you have eaten enough. Both protein and fat stimulate the release of leptin, which sends an "I'm full" (satiety) signal to the brain.[315] Carbohydrates are less likely to stimulate higher leptin levels while simultaneously engaging the pleasure center of the brain with endorphins, much like addictive drugs and alcohol.[316] While increased leptin means that we are less likely to eat protein or fat beyond satiation, there are no such controls for carbohydrate consumption. In fact, the opposite is true, resulting in a compulsion to continue eating carbohydrates despite the health dangers. The natural human tendency to overeat carbohydrates led to the concept of calorie restriction. In the long run, though, a conscious decision to limit calories is no match for hormonal impulses. We began counting our total calories when we should have been counting our total carbohydrates.

The Proper Healthy Human Diet: The Basics

Dr. Ken Berry is a family physician in Camden, Tennessee who, after managing his own obesity, prediabetes and severe reflux with a low-carbohydrate diet, began educating his patients on this way of eating as well. Dr Berry began using the phrase "the proper human diet" and now has a nutrition conference by the same name. This label is perfectly descriptive of a well-formulated ketogenic diet. *Proper* is defined as genuine, appropriate and suitable. I believe that an eating plan that keeps carbohydrates low while emphasizing protein, and the fat that naturally comes with it, is a diet that is most appropriate for humans. I have added the adjective *healthy* to promote healthy fats and animal-sourced foods.

What does a well-formulated ketogenic diet look like?

Carbohydrate Restriction.

A well-formulated ketogenic diet is less about what you should eat and more about what you don't eat. Carbohydrate consumption must be limited to 20 grams per day or less. This means avoiding all of the highest carbohydrate foods completely, including anything made with flour or sugar (bread, pasta, muffins, bagels, cake, candy, sugary beverages, fruit juices, etc.). Focus on low carbohydrate foods like non-starchy vegetables, leafy greens, dairy, eggs, fish and meats. When grocery shopping, stay at the perimeter of the store to focus on the butcher counter, the produce section, and the dairy cooler. The interior of the store is mainly stocked with packaged, highly processed, high-carbohydrate foods. See Appendix I for a great grocery list of low or no carbohydrate foods.

The metabolic theory of weight gain tells us that the presence of insulin stops fat burning for energy and instead promotes fat storage.[317] When we eat a diet high in carbohydrates, insulin is released to move glucose from the bloodstream into our cells. Blood sugar may drop well below baseline (see Figure 23), leading to desperate hunger and

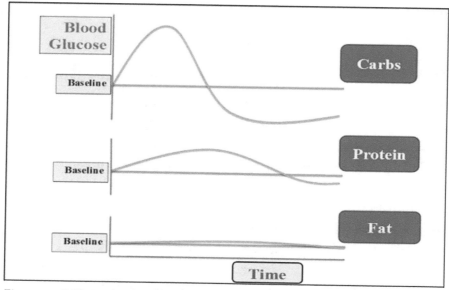

Figure 23. Differing levels of glucose in the blood in response to intake of the three macronutrients. Blood sugar rises the most with ingestion of carbohydrates. After a strong insulin response, glucose levels drop well below baseline inducing hunger, irritability, and weakness. In contrast, intake of protein results in a modest increase in glucose, while fat does not raise blood glucose levels at all.

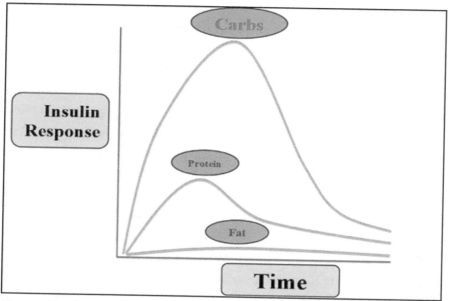

Figure 24. Insulin response to the three macronutrients. Carbohydrates elicit a very strong insulin response, proteins a moderate response, and fats very little or no insulin response.

the inclination to eat more carbohydrates. Because blood sugar does not rise as much, or at all, with ingestion of proteins or fats, there is a lowered insulin response and thus a decreased tendency to store fat.

The easiest way to avoid carbohydrates is to eat real food. Dr Robert Cywes, self-styled Carb Addiction Doc, has a great way of thinking about this. He maintains that "carbohydrates are not real food," and I would agree with him. Carbohydrates may be food for other animals, but they are not real food for humans. There are no essential carbohydrates, meaning humans don't need to eat them at all. Anytime we consume carbohydrates, it is purely for the addictive stimulation provided to the pleasure center of the brain.[318] When you think about carbohydrates in this way, it is easier to avoid consuming them.

Power of Sugar Addiction

My partner's roommate from college (let's call him Ken) would "sleep eat." Typically, the night after grocery shopping, Ken would walk into the kitchen while sound asleep, and devour a whole carton of ice cream and maybe some cookies. The next day, he would have no recollection of having done so. His wife had a lock put on the refrigerator and the key was given to their son, to be hidden. Ken would beg or try to bribe his son to give him the key. Sugar is a powerful and addictive substance!

Eat Enough Protein.

How much protein should be consumed? The optimal dietary protein intake has been analyzed for over a century[319] and there continues to be a great deal of controversy. The Recommended Daily Allowance (RDA) for protein, when reported as a percentage of calories, is such a large range (10 – 35 percent of calories), that it really offers very little guidance. The issue is further complicated because optimal levels of protein can change depending on age, health status, and level of activity. A burly ditch-digger generally needs way more protein than a petite, sedentary woman in her eighties.

Drs. Stephen Phinney and Jeff Volek, who have engaged in extensive research on healthy human diets for decades, suggest a range of protein intake between 1.5 and 2.0 grams of protein per kilogram of ideal body weight according to the Metropolitan Life tables (1959).[320] This means for a person whose ideal weight is 150 pounds (68 kg), the range for protein intake would be 102 to 138 grams per day. Intake may be on the higher end of the range when healing from the trauma of surgery or injury, recovering from an infection, if over the age of 70, or if regularly participating in intense exercise. Sometimes, the lower end of the range may be useful on the recommendation of a physician due to a medical condition such as hyperinsulinemia (high insulin in the blood).

There is a persistent myth that too much protein is hard on the kidneys, but several researchers have concluded that there is no evidence that eating excessive protein is harmful to healthy kidneys.[305,308] In a well-known experiment, two Arctic explorers were studied at Bellevue Hospital in New York for one year while they ate an all-meat diet. They were closely monitored by medical staff. No harm was found to their kidneys which continued to exhibit normal function.[286]

Because protein stimulates the release of leptin, the hormone that signals satiation, overconsuming protein is less of an issue. Dr. Ted Naiman, family medicine specialist and author of *The P:E Diet*, declares that people are compelled to eat continuously until they get enough protein.[321] This is a natural urge. A diet high in carbohydrates, or even fat, but low in protein will never quite satisfy this biological imperative and is one of the drivers of constant snacking, or grazing, across all waking hours.

Eat Fat to Satiation.

It would be quite difficult to consume too much fat as long as it is in its natural form and is a fat your body has evolved to consume. Be cautious, however, of drinking your energy. That is, I don't advocate such things as butter added to your coffee. If you like to drink coffee with added butter or coconut oil because you enjoy the taste, a bit won't hurt you, but don't try to get your "allotment" of fats in liquid form. Fat consumption should fulfill your energy needs and increase the palatability and texture of your food. Listen to your body and avoid overeating fat.

Good fats include primarily monounsaturated and saturated fatty acids, such as egg yolk, butter, olive oil, lard, beef tallow, cream, coconut oil and the essential polyunsaturated fats found principally in fish and shellfish (see Ketogenic Food List in Appendix I). Avoid industrialized seed and vegetable oils such as canola, corn and soybean oils. These polyunsaturated oils, highly processed with heat and chemicals, can create inflammation, and consequently swelling, in the body.[322] Saturated fat, conversely, is very stable and less likely to become rancid. A review of the available research completed over 20 years ago showed no association between cardiovascular disease and a diet high in saturated fats.[323] Despite ubiquitous diet recommendations to the contrary, saturated fats are healthy fats and favor a healthy lymphatic system.[324]

Ketosis and Ketones

What is ketosis? Ketones and fat, as well as glucose, can be used for energy. All human bodies produce ketones in response to a lack of carbohydrates or a lack of food (fasting). The blood levels of ketones produced is a function of the level of fat oxidation (burning). As carbohydrate intake is reduced or fasting is prolonged, insulin levels in the blood drop, and the rate of fat burning and ketone production increases. This is called "being in ketosis." Ketone levels in the blood can vary depending on diet, time of day, activity level, and other biochemical inputs, but the general goal of ketogenic nutrition is to become a "fat burner" in Dr. Eric Westman's lexicon.

Well-Formulated Ketogenic Diet Take-Aways

The simplicity of a ketogenic lifestyle can mean the freedom to prepare meals without drudgery, to eat luxurious foods without guilt, to occupy your time and mind without the distraction of carb addiction, and to enjoy your life without undue anxiety about your health. What follows are a few guiding principles to assist you in your ketogenic journey. Allow yourself to rethink what is accepted as the proper way to eat. As Jane Austen cogently says in *Emma*, *"What is right to be done cannot be done too soon."* Understanding these few recommendations will get you off on a good footing in your goal to create a healthier lymphatic system that will benefit you in ways you'd never imagine.

Eat Real Food.

For the most part, meals should be made up of whole foods with as little processing as possible. We have been trained to believe that the convenience of prepared, packaged meals is faster, less work, and just as healthy as a home cooked meal. Unfortunately, many of the additives and preservatives that allow that package to spend extended time on the shelf in the grocery store and later in the home pantry, create inflammation and are a burden on the lymphatic system. Meals should be composed of meats, poultry, fish, dairy, non-starchy vegetables, and leafy greens according to tolerances and preferences. Everything else is needless unhealthy filler.

Avoid Snacking.

The surest way to have a weight loss stall, re-awaken cravings, and possibly create undue inflammation is to revert to the SAD manner of eating: constant grazing and snacking. According to Carb Addiction Doc Robert Cywes, snacking is never a nutritional event. Instead, it is always an emotional one. If you are truly experiencing hunger, sit for an entire meal.

Eat When Hungry and Stop When Full.

Many people have grown up with the expectation of three meals per day that are eaten at certain times, whether or not we are hungry. The repetitiveness of the daily routine soon makes us actually feel hunger just prior to the expected eating time because the body learns to secrete the hunger hormone ghrelin in anticipation of the regularly occurring eating event.[325] When enjoying a ketogenic lifestyle, meal times are not always regimented, but follow in response to genuine body signals. You may find that your first meal is much later in the day because you don't wake up feeling hungry. Eating frequency and meal size may eventually drop off and a new routine will assert itself. Allow your body to guide you.

Stay Away From Sweeteners (Real Or Artificial).

When first transitioning to a sugar-restricted diet, it is not unusual to want to continue to enjoy sweet tasting foods. Many keto beginners will use sugar substitutes in the early stages. Carb Addiction Doc Robert Cywes supports the use of artificial sweeteners initially as a bridge to eventually giving up all sugar and sweeteners. If all sweet flavors are eliminated on the first day of the diet, Dr. Cywes believes this may prevent some people from even attempting a ketogenic lifestyle and realizing its benefits. Complete abstention, however, will be the eventual goal.

The perception of sweetness from artificial sweeteners can confuse your endocrine system and cause an insulin release because the taste and smell of sweetness sends a signal to the pancreas signaling the imminent need for insulin.[326] Since insulin promotes fat storage and stops fat burning, continued use of sweeteners could result in a weight loss stall. Additionally, regular consumption of sweet tasting foods can keep sugar cravings alive and make it a challenge to adhere to a ketogenic lifestyle particularly when exposed to favorite desserts. The best thing to do is get any and all sweeteners out of your pantry.

Avoid High Sugar Fruits.

An apple a day will keep the doctor away? Not really. Fruits are nature's candy. They contain a lot of carbs and can quickly take you out of fat-burning mode. Generally, the larger the fruit, the higher it is in carbohydrates. Berries are your best low carb choice but only as an occasional treat. (See the Ketogenic Food List in Appendix I). Flavor and a bit of sweetness can be had from a twist of lemon or lime in a beverage. An occasional dessert of berries, nuts and cream can provide you with some sweetness at the end of a meal but eventually you want to avoid fruit as much as possible for the same reasons that we avoid artificial sweeteners.

Your taste will soon become more sensitive and you will wonder how you ever tolerated the overly-sweetened foods that have become habitual in most Western diets. One study found that increased perception of sweetness occurred after just one month of reduced sugar intake. When given the choice to revert to their original level of sugar consumption, most participants in this study chose not to revert.[327] Beware of vegetables such as carrots and onions that turn sweet when you cook them. Ever wonder why sauteed onions are so sweet? It's all of that caramelized sugar.

Salt Your Food To Taste.

Sodium is a vital electrolyte that is essential for life. Yet we have been admonished to limit our salt intake to, as it turns out, dangerously low levels. Sodium performs many important roles in the body. These roles include fighting infection, facilitating muscle contraction and nerve cell transmission, regulating blood volume and maintaining the fluid balance in the tissues. Emergency room admissions, particularly for the elderly, for low levels of sodium in the blood are more than 31 times more frequent than admissions for too much sodium in the blood.[328] Low sodium is often the culprit in another common emergency room admission: heat stroke or heat exhaustion, during particularly hot weather. A vast amount of electrolytes, including sodium, may be lost from sweating, thus triggering these serious maladies if levels are not quickly replenished.

Most people who have a lymphatic disorder have been directed to severely limit their salt intake.[329] Certainly, anyone who eats a typical Western diet may even have noticed increased swelling whenever salty food is eaten. This is because a diet high in carbohydrates causes sodium retention, possibly due to the action of insulin,[330] so typical salty foods like potato chips and pretzels may indeed cause or exacerbate swelling. Conversely, when enjoying a ketogenic lifestyle, insulin remains at lower levels and sodium excretion in the urine is promoted. For this reason, eating a low-carbohydrate diet creates an even greater need for salt in the diet.[331]

Drs. John and Judith Casley-Smith, in their premier text about lymphedema and its treatment, are very explicit about "the uselessness of a low salt diet" for lymphedema management.[10] They specifically state that the common advice for people with a lymphatic disorder to adhere to a low salt or salt-free diet is as bad as prescribing diuretics (water pills) and has led to many people suffering needlessly from salt depletion. Ironically, low sodium can cause water retention and swelling, exactly the symptom that is being poorly managed with diuretics.

It is not uncommon for someone trained to limit their salt intake to experience flu-like symptoms in the first few weeks of adopting a ketogenic way of eating. Symptoms may include a headache, difficulty thinking, severe fatigue, irritability, and nausea. This so-called "keto flu" is often actually due to sodium depletion and can be remedied very quickly by ingesting some salt. When transitioning to a ketogenic way of eating, salting food to taste and drinking heated water with bouillon twice a day will help to maintain healthy levels of sodium in the body. Another favorite is eating pickles or drinking pickle juice. Please be aware, however, that several rare conditions may cause reduced tolerance for salt such as hyperaldosteronism, Cushing's disease and Liddle syndrome. It is wise to consult with a medical provider before altering your salt intake.

Eat Like a Rich Person.

Of all the factors that can sway dietary choices, affluence may have one of the biggest impacts. Would you think a rich person would add more noodles to extend a main dish? Or is it more likely that langoustine and saffron would be added to their bouillabaisse?

Health and longevity seem to track closely with income. In one study, the increase in life expectancy grew fifteen years for men and ten years for women as income increased.[332] Many reasons could account for this, including differences in medical care access, housing circumstances, labor market conditions such as unemployment rates, and health behaviors such as smoking and exercise.

But what is the impact of wealth on diet? I believe that the wealthier they are, the better people eat. When people have ability and access, largely due to their income, they will choose the healthier option more often than not.[333] In one study, people with lower incomes were more likely to purchase sweets, packaged snacks, frozen desserts, and sugar sweetened beverages. They were less inclined to purchase dairy products or seafood.[334] In this same study, almost 80 percent of the low-income participants were obese while 30 percent of their wealthier counterparts were. Members of households with food insecurity and lower nutrient intake are more at risk for a wide range of health conditions such as anemia, diabetes, hypertension, obesity, and sleep disturbances[335] all of which can have a negative impact on the lymphatic system.

It is a well-studied phenomenon that poor neighborhoods are plagued by what has been termed food deserts, areas dominated by stores offering little besides high-carbohydrate, high-sugar, non-nutritious packaged food-like substances.[336] Carbohydrates, the cheapest ingredients that can be added to food products, make up the majority of the foods available and consumed in these impoverished areas, a situation that negatively affects the health of the populace unlucky enough to be living there. Areas populated by rich people, in contrast, have many options for nutritious food, including frequent farmers' markets, and grocery stores offering an almost unimaginable variety of excellent, high quality foods from around the world. When money is no object, the choices tend more toward meat, delicacies, and high quality vegetables.

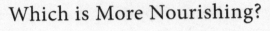

Which is More Nourishing?

This? Healthy fats, protein and micronutrient-rich.   *Or this? Mostly carbohydrates, almost no micronutrients, fat or protein.*

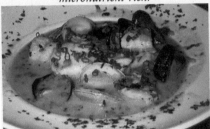 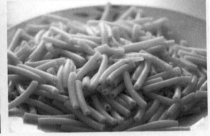

Furthermore, which one is a poor person more likely to eat?

But is it really more expensive to eat healthy? Certainly many carbohydrate-heavy packaged foods are cheaper to produce and have a longer shelf life than fresh meats, dairy and produce. But several factors may make a well-formulated ketogenic diet a substantially less expensive eating plan. Because protein and fat are more nutrient dense than carbohydrate-heavy foods, meals are smaller and less frequent (sometimes just once or twice a day). In this case, although some individual foods may be more expensive, someone on a well-formulated ketogenic diet will consume less of them. Expensive packaged snacks become a thing of the past because hunger between meals is overcome. Starches and sugars (carbohydrates) are the major contributors to frequent hunger. Even though one may be eating more volume when eating carbohydrates, the effect on insulin and blood sugar will lead to constant hunger, the result of which is buying more food, leading to a never-ending cycle of hunger and eating. This is the trap of high-carbohydrate consumption seen in the SAD and plant-based diets (see Figure 26 on next page).

Perhaps the greatest cost-saving measure of a ketogenic eating plan is the reduced medication and healthcare bills realized when your health is better managed. Continuing to eat a predominantly plant-based, high-carbohydrate diet is likely to lead to serious medical conditions, impaired lymphatic function, loss of income, loss of independence, and shorter lifespan. Now, that is expensive. So, pretend you are well-to-do. Eat like a rich person and you'll enhance your health and lymphatic system and you will become rich in so many ways. (See Making Keto Fit Your Budget in Appendix IV of this book for further cost-effective suggestions.)

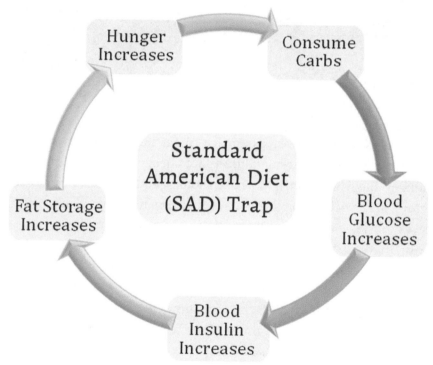

Figure 26. The Standard American Diet (SAD) traps people in this vicious carbohydrate cycle. Intake of carbohydrates causes blood sugar to increase and induces the release of insulin. Insulin immediately stops fat burning and encourages fat storage, while triggering hunger because blood sugar has dropped so low. This prompts the intake of more carbs. (Adapted from a presentation by Dr. Sarah Hallberg).

With a better understanding of the nuts and bolts of a ketogenic diet, we can turn to common issues and challenges that may be encountered when adopting a ketogenic diet. In the next chapter, I examine issues that could pose challenges, like making adaptations for previous weight loss surgery, fighting carb addiction, or overcoming the fear of eating fat. The challenges are not insurmountable, because knowledge is power, and it can help you plan for success.

Chapter 7

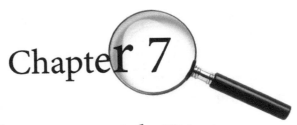

Special Issues with Dietary Change

"You know my methods. Apply them."
—*Arthur Conan Doyle, The Sign of The Four*

In this chapter, I will discuss several common issues and challenges associated with adopting a ketogenic diet. You may breeze through your transition to a ketogenic way of eating and never experience any of the issues listed here. My goal is to inform you so that, having been forewarned, you can avoid pitfalls or unpleasant experiences. Once informed, you may also be able to advise someone else who is struggling with dietary change due to unexpected consequences. Lastly, I hope to dispel any misgivings that may be associated with having a lymphatic disorder and explain the special issues that may come up for you. As always, it is recommended that you enlist a healthcare provider who is familiar with your unique situation and medical history to monitor and guide you, so that you have support if any distressing symptoms arise.

Electrolyte Imbalance

One of the main reasons that people experience ill-effects while on a ketogenic diet is because they aren't replenishing their electrolytes as they limit their carbohydrates. Electrolytes are electrically charged particles that are important for managing fluid and pH balance in the body and are vital for muscle contraction. The most important electrolytes are sodium, calcium, potassium, and magnesium.

Carbohydrate restriction changes the way that water and electrolytes are handled in the body. When eating a high-carbohydrate diet, energy is stored in muscles as glycogen, a process which requires a large amount of water.[337] In the first weeks of limited carbohydrate intake, glycogen storage is reduced and water is released, accounting for the majority of initial weight loss.[338] Additionally, insulin is known to cause sodium and potassium retention. A reduction of carbohydrate intake will mean lower insulin levels and an increase in electrolyte excretion.[339]

Because electrolytes follow the water, symptoms of electrolyte depletion can appear. These can include headaches, dizziness, confusion, fatigue, muscle cramping and weakness, and even nausea and vomiting. Because of the similarity of symptoms with the flu, people who experience this are said to be suffering from "keto flu." Hence, replenishing electrolytes daily will keep you feeling energized and healthy. The list below is meant to be a guide to help you do that. Additionally, establishing electrolyte levels with a blood test can help you and your medical provider determine if electrolyte supplementation is needed.

- **Sodium:** As discussed in Chapter 6, despite conventional recommendations for low salt intake when diagnosed with a lymphatic disorder, demands for sodium will be even higher when on a ketogenic eating plan. Some medical conditions may require salt restriction, so consult your healthcare provider before increasing your salt intake.

- **Calcium:** Many of the foods recommended on a ketogenic diet (i.e., dark leafy greens, cheeses, canned fish with bones, and nuts) provide ample amounts of calcium. Because the use of calcium supplementation has been associated with cardiovascular risk, it is preferred to get calcium from these whole foods rather than from pills. [340] Getting adequate levels of vitamins D (found in meats, poultry, egg yolk, and mushrooms) and K_2 (found in pastured eggs, liver and some cheeses) will enhance the absorption of calcium.[341] Ask your healthcare provider if you should be taking Vitamin D and/or K_2 supplements along with eating foods high in calcium and these vitamins.

- **Potassium:** This electrolyte is plentiful in ketogenic foods such as avocados, mushrooms, green leafy vegetables, and meat. Because high blood levels of potassium can be dangerous, only use a potassium supplement under the direction of your doctor.

- **Magnesium:** Foods such as dark leafy greens, avocado, halibut, salmon, mackerel, chicken and beef are rich in magnesium. Because most people tend to be low in magnesium, and this electrolyte is known to help with constipation and sleep, many people new to a ketogenic lifestyle would benefit from using a magnesium supplement. Magnesium citrate tends to be more easily absorbed and the daily recommended intake is 300-400 mg/day.[342]

Gastrointestinal Distress

Making a radical change in diet, even a healthy change, can initially cause some gastrointestinal distress such as constipation or diarrhea. Part of the reason is that our intestinal microbiome (the resident microorganisms in our gut) become suited to the foods that we typically eat. A diet composed primarily of chicken nuggets, French fries, and milkshakes will support a completely different set of gut microbes than one composed of fresh fish, eggs, and beef.[343,344] A disruption to normal dietary habits may cause some distress until new gut microbes can move in.

Your lower intestinal tract is a creature of habit, preferring to have the same foods at the same time and even to use the same toilet. This is most obvious with a phenomenon known as "travel constipation".[345] We are often exposed to different foods as well as time changes and potentially less access to a bathroom when traveling, and these changes can contribute to temporary constipation. This may happen with a change in dietary habits as well. Dr. Eric Westman, a ketogenic diet expert at Duke University's Keto Medicine Clinic, recommends milk of magnesia for the constipation that may appear when first transitioning to a ketogenic eating plan.[346]

Diarrhea is less common but can still be related to dietary change or to other health concerns and conditions. Gallbladder removal and some types of weight loss surgery can cause diarrhea in response to eating fat. These issues will be discussed later in this chapter. Other causes of diarrhea may be stomach flu, gastrointestinal disease, medication reaction, or stress, and should all be ruled out by your medical provider, even if the onset seems to correspond to the timing of a change in your diet.

Food Boredom

Occasionally I have heard from clients and others who say that they would find eating bacon and eggs every morning boring. This complaint is odd as often these same people have told me that they have started each day for the past thirty years or so with cereal or waffles. Certainly, you don't have to eat the same thing each day on a ketogenic eating plan. There are innumerable foods that fit a ketogenic lifestyle. A morning meal can include fish, fowl, meat, low starch vegetables, or unsweetened fruit such as olives, avocado, and cucumber. In fact, it's an opportunity to consider eating something that isn't traditionally considered a breakfast food. Feel like having a big juicy steak? Go for it! Salmon with a delicious cream sauce? Have at it! Many people have found that they like routine and will eventually settle on the same few items for every meal. That's also no problem. Keep your carbohydrate intake below 20 grams a day and eat when hungry, stop when full.

Social Eating

Along with food boredom, many people say they would not enjoy going to restaurants or to social affairs if they cannot have what is standard fare on the menu or what others in the gathering are enjoying. This may be an indication that food is being used to entertain. An alternative way to consider social outings is to place more value on the conversation and comradery enjoyed with dining companions. Food, although it can be enjoyable, is for sustenance, not entertainment. In other words, when food is the focus, the social aspect becomes secondary, and family and friends rank below that focus. There are too many other things in life to appreciate. Don't put food at the top of that list.

When one low-carb physician was asked how he could celebrate if he didn't eat traditional celebratory foods like cake, he replied, "I kiss my wife!" Consider all of the non-food methods you can use to celebrate, such as a hug or high five, singing, dancing, and enjoyment of fellowship.

In addition, many people find it difficult to make good choices in a restaurant or social setting. They may fear questions about their choices or being seen as different. And often, social situations offer sparse ketogenic options. It takes courage to take care of yourself. Here are a few tips to help you navigate social situations that will include food:

- Defensive eating. Eat a nice ketogenic meal before the social event. You will be less inclined to give in to temptation if you aren't hungry.

- Offer to contribute something so you know there will be something you can eat.

- Have a ready explanation for your food choices and/or refusals that you feel comfortable with. For example:
  - » "I'm testing to see if I'm allergic to (chocolate, dairy, sugar, wheat, etc) so I can't have that right now."
  - » "I've started a special way of eating and have already lost XX pounds, so I don't want to quit now. I know you'll support me on this!"
  - » "My doctor has put me on a special diet."

- Fill your plate up with foods you can eat. A full plate isn't as obvious as one that has very little on it.

- Let your host know of your food restrictions ahead of time and ask what will be served. If forewarned, the cook should not be offended if you decline certain dishes.

- You don't have to offer any explanation if you aren't asked.

Restaurant Strategies

Have some restaurant strategies ready:

- Read the restaurant menu ahead of time and make your selections.

- Order one meal and split it between two people.

- Can you make substitutions? Order extra veggies instead of baked potato or bread.

- Ask if wheat flour is used to make sauces or soups.

- Ask for extra butter, no bread.

- Ask for olive oil.

- Avoid anything that is "breaded."

- If a dish is "stuffed," ask what is in the stuffing.

- Avoid dishes labeled "gluten-free." They are generally made with another carb such as corn, potato or tapioca starch.

- You can also "eat around the carbs." For example, ignore the red potatoes and just eat the green beans.

Some Additional Fast Food Strategies

- Ask for a lettuce wrap or have the burger served on a bed of lettuce. One fast food chain calls this "protein style."

- Eat the toppings off the pizza and throw away the crust.

- Avoid French fries and soda. Substitute side salad and unsweetened iced tea.

- Open up the taco or burrito and just eat the insides.

- Think of the bun, tortilla, and crust as the plate delivering the good stuff. Don't eat the plate!

- Avoid fried chicken at fast food restaurants. The breading is not keto, and these foods are usually deep fried in vegetable oils, which easily go rancid and are not healthy.

Bariatric Surgery

Weight-loss surgery has seen a stunning rise in popularity in the United States over the last two decades. In 1998, approximately 13,000 bariatric surgeries were performed in the US.[347] By 2018, this number had climbed to 228,000 (American Society for Metabolic and Bariatric Surgery, 2018). One of the drivers of this surge was early research which suggested weight loss surgery, particularly the Roux-en-Y, could reverse Type 2 diabetes. But more recent research has revealed that the pre-surgery very-low-calorie diet (and inevitable reduction in carbohydrate consumption) was responsible instead.[348]

Regardless, the large amount of weight that can be lost in a short amount of time, as well as other possible health benefits are compelling reasons for this stampede toward the operating table. Reports of losing over 100 pounds in less than a year and the possible resolution of chronic weight-related diseases make going under the knife even more alluring.[347] Add to this the very real desperation of people who have unsuccessfully struggled with weight loss for most of their lives and you can understand the appeal. It's frustrating, disheartening and frightening to live with obesity and life-threatening chronic disease. In one study, the most common reasons cited for seeking weight loss surgery were related to health and the fear of early death.[349] Most studies show an improvement in quality of life in those who undergo surgery, at least in the short term.[350]

Unfortunately, there are many possible lifelong side effects to weight-loss surgeries that might discourage some from choosing this option.[351] The research literature reports weight regain, nutritional deficiencies, various complications requiring further surgery, dumping syndrome, hair loss, infection, bowel obstruction, acid reflux, increased incidence of alcohol abuse, and increased risk of death from all causes among the consequences of bariatric surgery.[347,352–356]

In their 2021 updated Obesity Algorithm document, the Obesity Medicine Association (OMA) cites additional serious "acute complications" such as gastrointestinal obstruction and bleeding, pneumonia, blood clots, pulmonary embolism, and death. Their list of long term difficulties includes gallstones, hyperparathyroidism, small intestine bacterial overgrowth, kidney stones, anemia, neuropathy, osteoporosis, and depression. Yet, given the potential risks of severe obesity, many people still elect to have weight-loss surgery regardless of this catalog of significant common hazards. Thus is the stigma and misery of being obese.

Can a ketogenic diet be followed by those who have already had weight-loss surgery? The answer is yes, and in fact, a ketogenic diet may be particularly suited for someone who has undergone one of these procedures. In order to explain how, we first need to explore the various types of weight-loss surgeries.

There are two main ways that bariatric surgeries work: restriction and malabsorption. Restriction means that the amount of food the stomach is able to hold is reduced. Alternatively, nutrients are prevented from being absorbed or used by the body in surgical techniques that feature malabsorption. Some procedures, like the Roux-en-Y gastric bypass (RNY), use both restriction and malabsorption. Some bariatric procedures such as gastric band or balloon can be temporary, and might later be removed, restoring the stomach to normal function. Others, like the RNY, are permanent and non-reversible. Once the stomach or intestines are partially removed, they cannot be retrieved, and patients will spend the rest of their lives trying to duplicate the vital functions these healthy body parts had once performed so effortlessly.

Essentially, resecting healthy tissue is not a viable solution long-term. There is no other condition besides obesity that offers surgery on normal, properly functioning tissue to fix that condition. A nutritional problem cannot be corrected with a surgical fix. But once surgery has taken place, how best can health and quality of life be pursued?

Post-surgery diet recommendations are similar across the board for most weight-loss surgeries, but tragically many of the suggestions are not backed up by science or research. Generally, recommendations include: eating up to six small meals per day, chewing food thoroughly, restricting fat intake, limiting fluid intake with meals, and including vitamin/mineral supplementation. Eating high amounts of protein is suggested for improving healing from surgery. Because simple carbohydrates are known to cause dumping syndrome, a potentially severe gastrointestinal condition that can occur after surgical weight loss procedures, foods like white bread and anything "obviously full of sugar like candy, ice cream or donuts"[357] should be avoided. Additionally, patients are generally advised to eat mostly so-called "nutrient-dense vegetables."

An eating plan should provide essential nutrients in amounts that promote healing and recovery, health, satiation, and a good quality of life. All of these needs can be met most effectively with a well-formulated ketogenic diet. It can be suitable for most people as soon as solid food is allowed immediately post-surgery and can be crucial in aiding recovery and healing. Some bariatric procedures, such as biliopancreatic diversion with a duodenal switch (BPD-DS) and RNY, result in the poor absorption of fat and subsequent diarrhea,[358,359] requiring a lower consumption of this macronutrient and medical supervision. But most bariatric procedures do not require a limit on dietary fat. Furthermore, in the initial stages of adopting a ketogenic diet, eating a high amount of fat may not be essential, especially in the case of obesity. "An obese person can get all the fat they need for a ketogenic diet by using their own body fat stores," stated Dr. Eric Westman, during my 2014 visit to the Duke University Keto Medicine Clinic in Durham, NC.

As discussed earlier, dumping syndrome is most often a reaction to eating simple carbohydrates. Symptoms may include "facial flushing, lightheadedness, fatigue, reactive hypoglycemia, and postprandial diarrhea." According to the OMA,[360] dumping syndrome is a "unique complication of RNY" and "occurs in approximately 70-85 percent of [these] patients." Both types of this complication, early and late dumping, can be completely avoided on a ketogenic diet because carbohydrates are severely restricted. Advice to eat nutrient dense foods after bariatric surgery is fine advice, and easily accomplished with ketogenic nutrition, as well.

Another advantage to following a ketogenic diet has to do with portion control. Since the size of the stomach is much smaller after surgery, it is important to choose foods with the most nutrients possible to fill that smaller space. As discussed in Chapter 6, food portions in ketogenic meals are much smaller due to the higher density and bioavailability of nutrients found in foods included in this way of eating. In fact, because of the improved nutrient bioavailability from animal-sourced foods, a well-formulated ketogenic diet can also aid with vitamin and mineral deficiencies which are commonly experienced following many weight loss procedures.

About one half of all bariatric surgery patients regain up to 40 percent of their excess weight within the first two years.[361] This is most likely because patients continue to eat a high-carbohydrate Standard American Diet after surgery. Even though meals are much smaller than before surgery, the same body mechanisms that enhanced fat storage and blocked fat burning continue to hold sway after surgery. The very disheartening and common eventual outcome of weight regain can be effectively eliminated by adopting a well-formulated ketogenic diet.

Gallstones and Gallbladder Surgery

The gallbladder is a small pouch that stores bile and then releases it into the small intestine in response to the presence of dietary fat. Bile is necessary for fat digestion and absorption.

The most common affliction of the gallbladder is gallstones, which can become quite painful when a stone becomes lodged in the common bile duct. Prevailing medical wisdom has blamed the increased concentration of certain substances associated with obesity, such as cholesterol, as well as diets high in sugar and fat for the formation of painful gallstones.[362] A large body of research, however, also points to adherence to a very low-calorie, low-fat diet and/or the rapid weight loss associated with bariatric surgeries as the more likely culprits.[363–365] There exists such a high risk of gallstones with rapid weight loss that some have suggested removing the gallbladder at the time of bariatric surgery.[366]

There seems to be a lot of agreement in the medical literature that the best method to prevent gallstone formation is by eating a high fat diet.[364,367] Why would a high-fat diet be better than a low-fat diet? The gallbladder's function is to release bile when fat enters the digestive tract. If a person is following a low-fat diet, there's no fat trigger to nudge the gallbladder to act, so the bile isn't excreted. Bile is made up of mineral salts, and if you have ever dumped salt into a glass of water, you know it won't mix with the water until you stir it vigorously. It's the same with bile. The mineral salts in the bile settle out if they aren't mixed, and as they clump together, stones are more likely to form.

But there's a caveat. Although a high-fat diet may prevent gallstone formation, once stones are already present, changing to a diet high in fat may actually bring on an attack. When the gallbladder contracts to release bile in response to dietary fat, any stones formed while it sat idle may then be pushed into the common bile duct. A stone lodged in the duct is the cause of the incredible pain associated with a gallbladder attack. But it is also possible that an attack might be avoided because any stones present could end up passing through without getting caught in the duct. In this way, the stones can be flushed out of the gallbladder due to the more constant need for bile with a high-fat diet. If you have a history of gallstones, gradually increasing your intake of fat may be the best option. Consultation with a nutritionist who is familiar with gallstones and a ketogenic diet may also be helpful.

Even after gallbladder removal, it is still possible to eat a well-formulated ketogenic diet. Instead of releasing stored bile in response to the intake of dietary fat, a little bit of bile is released into the intestines continuously and may not be enough to adequately digest all the fat in a large meal. Ellen Davis, MS, a clinical nutritionist, offers these tips[368] if you would like to start a ketogenic diet after having your gallbladder removed:

» Increase your fat intake slowly.

» Eat smaller meals, which are more easily digested.

» Focus on fats that don't need bile to be digested (butter, coconut oil).

» Taking an ox bile salt supplement may help with fat digestion.

Carbohydrate Addiction

Carbohydrate addiction may be the single most powerful reason why most traditional weight-loss diets fail and it can make the early phase of adopting a ketogenic diet a struggle for many people. The concept of carbohydrate addiction is not new, merely forgotten by the current generation.[369,370] Lately, we have been reminded of what we used to know by physicians like Dr. Robert Cywes, who calls himself The Carb Addiction Doc (see links to his YouTube channel in Resources). Dr. Cywes explains that carbohydrate, like alcohol, is a non-essential nutrient that can very strongly activate the endorphin system. Carbohydrates can give us instant pleasure, euphoria, and calm, but those good feelings come with a high price tag attached: ultimate psychological harm from addiction, guilt, and repression as well as physical harm from the damage of high levels of blood sugar and insulin resistance leading to a host of chronic illnesses.[370] I believe that physical harm is also being perpetrated on the lymphatic system by the inflammatory effects of carbohydrates.

Understanding homeostasis is important in the discussion of carbohydrate addiction. The human body strives to maintain a stable, relatively constant internal environment. Homeostasis is the balance that the body achieves by prompting actions to make adjustments through feedback mechanisms. Levels of all essential nutrients, vitamins, minerals and water are tightly controlled in the human body in this way. The body will send feedback that urges us to seek out or refuse an essential substance in order to maintain proper levels. We have no need to calculate how much sodium we need to have on a daily basis, for instance. If we are low in sodium, we experience symptoms such as light-headedness and fatigue as well as a craving for salty food. Too much sodium, on the other hand, triggers thirst. The feedback mechanism for sodium encourages an action that can help us maintain sodium homeostasis. Similar mechanisms exist for other essential nutrients like protein, fat and water.

As discussed in Chapter 6, carbohydrates are not essential and can not be considered food. Similar to alcohol, carbohydrates are consumed solely for the pleasure they provide and, also like alcohol, there is no feedback mechanism to signal when to stop eating them. On the contrary, the instant gratification by stimulation of endorphin pathways in the brain strongly encourages us not to stop. And because of the robust insulin response to carbohydrates, subsequent blood sugar levels drop well below baseline creating a horrible feeling of unease, weakness and tremendous hunger. The fear of this unpleasant and dangerous experience prompts almost constant grazing on more carbohydrates to prevent its recurrence.

Essentially, the concept of "calories" came about in an effort to artificially provide negative feedback to control the portion size when eating carbohydrates. However, because of the promotion of carbohydrates as a health food and the urging of our own biology to eat this nutrient excessively, we have conflated calorie counting to be necessary for all foods. This, of course, has translated into recommendations for very-low calorie diets that unfortunately continue to foster tremendous carbohydrate addiction and which are impossible to sustain.

How did we become addicted to carbohydrates? Availability may be one of the most compelling reasons. Early humans subsisted primarily on hunted foods that were only supplemented by plant foods when in season and necessary for survival.[371] Even with the advent of agriculture 10,000 years ago, carbohydrate consumption was not very high. A huge change happened during the Industrial Era, and to an even greater extent in the last one hundred years, when access to shelf-stable foods high in carbohydrates became available year-round almost anywhere in the world.[284] Once we learned that any stress or unpleasant emotion could be quickly assuaged by the easily available and cheap drug known as carbohydrates, it was a short walk to addiction. And when everyone around you is also addicted to these foods, it doesn't seem abnormal.

The substance abuse model can be useful to understand and circumvent carbohydrate addiction. Substance abuse is defined as using and continuing to use a substance to manage emotions to the point of harm. This concept can easily be applied to uncontrolled carbohydrate consumption despite harm to health. Dr. Cywes recommends that, like drug addiction, carbohydrate addiction requires complete abstinence and perhaps professional assistance to beat it. Health care providers and coaches versed in a ketogenic lifestyle may help monitor your health and optimize your outcomes by helping you combat carbohydrate addiction.

I feel compelled here to address the concept of "food addiction." The idea that humans can be considered to be addicted to something necessary for survival does not make sense to me. The proponents of this concept insist that they really mean "processed food addiction" and it is really just a point of semantics that we disagree on. First, words matter, and language needs to be concise to make sure we are properly understood. Second, processed food addiction is still not precise enough. Making brie cheese requires a complex production process but I don't believe this particular "processed food" inspires addiction. It seems that the real concern of the processed food addiction movement is the harmful additives, preservatives and heating/chemical processes used in many food products. Most of these foods happen to also be high in carbohydrate. I believe it is the carbohydrate that is actually addictive and harmful. And that harm is certainly greatly compounded by the chemical additives and high heat used in their manufacture.

Restricting Calories and Fasting

"Three days of absolute fast does not improve one's beauty, Watson."
Sir Arthur Conan Doyle, The Dying Detective

There is strong evidence that medically supervised fasting alternating with a ketogenic eating plan can be a potent complement to treatments for conditions such as epilepsy and cancer. However, all of the benefits of fasting, such as ketosis, autophagy, lower insulin levels, decreased blood pressure and more,[372] can also be achieved with a ketogenic eating plan. Many have speculated that the advantages of fasting may merely be that during a fast, fewer carbohydrates are consumed.[285]

Ketones are healthy metabolites of fat burning, and they are increased in the body by 1) a ketogenic way of eating, 2) fasting, or 3) starvation. A ketogenic eating plan has been previously defined and described in Chapter 5. Fasting is abstaining from food or drink for a prescribed amount of time. "Wet" fasting allows water and electrolytes while "dry" does not allow even this fluid intake. Starvation can be described as suffering and/or death due to insufficient food. While all of these methods will induce a state of ketosis (described in Chapter 6), only a ketogenic way of eating is sustainable indefinitely.

A ketogenic eating plan can also claim fewer adverse events along with similar therapeutic benefits to fasting, all without hunger, deprivation or suffering.[373,374] In actuality, fasting does not increase ketones any more than a well-formulated ketogenic diet does. In fact, at times, fasting can result in higher baseline blood sugars, which can increase insulin and lower ketone production. This is a phenomenon called physiological insulin resistance, in which the body uses fatty acids and ketones preferentially for muscle and cardiac function, leaving more glucose in the bloodstream for brain function. Exercise while fasting can also increase blood sugar for longer periods of time as muscle prefers to burn fatty acids for fuel. The bottom line is that the carbohydrate restriction observed on a ketogenic diet keeps blood glucose levels steady, allowing you to eat satiating, delicious food without hunger.

Amber O'Hearn, a respected Carnivore diet advocate, has stated her astonishment that even when the benefits of a ketogenic diet are known by nutrition experts, they have difficulty reconciling this knowledge with their deeply held belief that a healthy diet must necessarily be plant-based, low-fat, and high-carbohydrate. This is exemplified in the work of Valter Longo, an Italian-American scientist who is known for his animal studies on fasting. Using considerable mental gymnastics, he is able to promote an eating plan that disallows fat and red meat and requires frequent multi-day fasts in order to bring about the benefits of ketosis.

I am not a fan of fasting, although many women with lipedema use it and are somewhat successful with it. My worry is that life-long "dieters" have learned to associate hunger and a feeling of deprivation with weight loss success. We have trained ourselves to ignore body signals when doing traditional diets in order to lessen the suffering of a very low-calorie, low-fat diet. Looking at a clock to see if it is time to eat instead of sensing whether or not we are hungry, further distances us from grasping what our body is trying to tell us.

Sometimes it is a question of language. Technically, anytime you aren't eating, you are fasting. I like to simply call it *not eating*. In practice, "eat when you're hungry and stop when you're full" and "do a 16:8 intermittent fast" may both mean eating two meals per day, but the first maxim is listening to your body instead of artificially heeding the clock. For someone who has a history of disordered eating, fasting may accentuate that poor relationship with food by providing a false sense of power or control.

While there are some adverse effects of fasting noted in the medical literature, such as weight loss due predominantly to muscle loss[375] and the hazards of refeeding syndrome,[376] the adverse effects seem to be even worse with a long term low-calorie diet. This was most evident with the long term metabolic damage done to participants of the Biggest Loser weight loss television series.[239] The participants for the most part suffered moderate weight regain and persistent metabolic slowing, including a decreased resting metabolic rate and famine response hypothyroidism, six years after the competition. This is all compounded by the increased social stigma against obesity that was fostered by the program.[377] Prolonged low calorie diets have also been shown to increase the responsiveness of fat tissue to *lipoprotein lipase* (LPL), an enzyme that pulls fat into fat cells. In one study, women who had used an 800 calorie per day diet for three months showed a 12-fold increase in LPL activity.[378]

Starting and Stopping Keto

Living with a lymphatic or adipose tissue disorder requires sticking to a lifelong self-management program. Following a ketogenic lifestyle, just like wearing compression garments, will be integral to achieving and sustaining optimal outcomes. And like compression garments, your eating plan can be over-the-counter or prescription strength. Many people find that their lymphedema is better managed when they wear their custom flat knit compression garments on a daily basis just as they do best when faithfully adhering to a ketogenic lifestyle. Taking a day off keto or having a "cheat meal" occasionally is like taking a day off of wearing your compression garments or wearing cheap stockings from a drug store rather than well-fitting stockings specifically made for managing lymphedema. Give yourself the best chance possible of keeping your swelling down, reducing your risk of infection, managing your pain and more by adhering to your eating plan as strictly as possible.

Be aware that there are metabolic consequences for jumping off the wagon occasionally. What might those be? To answer this question, a few terms need to be defined. When dietary carbohydrates are reduced significantly to less than 50 grams per day, the body will begin producing more ketones. When ketone levels in the blood reach at least 0.5 millimolars per deciliter, you are said to be in *nutritional ketosis.* According to Drs. Jeff Volek and Stephen Phinney, it may take you anywhere from three days to one to two weeks to achieve this state. Ketosis is different from *fat adaptation.* When first restricting carbohydrate intake, you may experience some fatigue while your body searches for the missing fuel to which it has become accustomed. As a sugar-burner, your body will still look for sugar and may, for a time, convert protein to glucose (either dietary protein or proteins from your muscle) using an inefficient process called gluconeogenesis. Becoming *fat-adapted* means that your body has successfully adapted itself to efficiently metabolizing fat for fuel rather than carbohydrates. This process can take several months, particularly for someone with a compromised metabolism (type 2 diabetes) and/or a chronic condition (lymphedema/lipedema). If you get in the habit of stopping and starting a ketogenic eating plan, you'll have to go through the process of achieving nutritional ketosis and becoming fat-adapted each time.

Additionally, there is good evidence that eating high levels of carbohydrates, even in the short term (such as a "cheat meal"), causes harm to both the metabolism and the lymphatic system. Blood and lymphatic vessels become leaky when exposed to hyperglycemia (high blood sugar) which can result in increased swelling.[43,379] Consuming carbohydrates can also increase inflammation[380,381] which has been linked to pain, especially in lipedema.[382] Conversely, when you are in ketosis and fat-adapted, inflammation, pain and body fat are reduced. In addition, lymphatic vessels may use ketones preferentially to heal and produce more vessels.[28] In general, sticking to a ketogenic eating plan will be best for your lymphatic system and health overall.

Comparing Your Results With Others

Even though a ketogenic diet is beneficial for many health concerns, many people will focus solely on its proven effectiveness for weight loss. Quite often, the success of any diet is exclusively based on what the scale says. And the frustration of slow weight loss can be compounded by comparing your results to others who may appear to be shedding pounds effortlessly. It may even lead you to believe that you are experiencing a weight loss stall. Hence, it's important to remember the reasons why people vary in response to a ketogenic lifestyle.

There are many factors that can influence how quickly your weight changes.[383] For instance:

- Men tend to lose weight faster than women.
- Previous experience with repeated weight loss and weight regain may have slowed your metabolism.
- Medications can interfere with weight loss and also cause weight gain.
- Depending on the type, intensity and frequency of exercise, changes in bone density and muscle mass can account for lack of weight loss, since muscle tissue is heavier than fat tissue.

All or some of these barriers to weight loss may be at play in specific cases. And even though success is not seen on the scale, it may be quite evident in other ways. As I will discuss in Chapter 8, a ketogenic lifestyle allows healing, rejuvenation and a renewed vitality you may not have experienced before. This means that you will need to recognize multiple measures of success. Consider documenting changes in pain levels, waist measure, energy level, skin, hair and nail quality, and the fit of your clothes and compression garments. Has your doctor lowered the dosage or stopped some of your medications? Are you wearing a smaller clothing size? All of these signs of improvements in your health can be happening even if the scale isn't moving.

Jackie Eberstein, a nurse who worked with Dr. Robert Atkins (The Atkins Diet) for over thirty years, recommends that you have a *size* goal rather than a *weight* goal. What size would you like to be? What size of clothing would you like to wear? What would you like your waist measurement to be? If you have lymphedema, what size would you like the affected area of your body to be? Instead of comparing the results of your weight loss efforts with others, look for evidence of what is happening in your body and how these changes benefit you. More important than attaining a certain number on the scale is to lose fat, increase bone density and muscle mass, and improve metabolism and lymphatic function. Adhere to a well-formulated ketogenic diet and eventually your body will settle to a weight you will be comfortable with: the healthiest one.

Fear of Fat

"Convince a man against his will, He's of the same opinion still."
From notes to Chapter 5 of Mary Wollstonecraft's
1792 treatise, A Vindication of the Rights of Woman

A fear of eating fat can pose a challenge to adopting a ketogenic lifestyle. This is an unfortunate consequence of the USDA's Dietary Guideline's persistent and obstinate advice that "fat is bad." It has fostered an unhealthy anxiety in the collective American mind about the health implications of eating fat, especially animal fats. Although it is beyond the purview of this book to examine the moral and environmental issues surrounding a diet that is at least partially supplied by animal sources (see Resources for book and website recommendations for more information on this issue), I hope to at least address and allay the fears of readers who are unsure about the health implications of eating fats.

Many of us have grown up with the ideology that a healthy diet was one that had very little fat or animal-sourced foods. Getting most of your nutrition from plants was and still is revered. For decades, experts have advised the use of so-called "healthy" alternatives to animal-based foods, such as margarine instead of butter, seed oils instead of lard, and fake meats made out of soy. This irrationality started in the mid-19th century most notably by John Harvey Kellogg, inventor of Kellogg's cereals and temperance health reformer. He promoted religious admonitions to give up all vices, such as alcohol, tobacco, caffeine and meat.[384] The first nutrition education programs, as well as the establishment of the American Dietetics Association, were founded on vegetarian beliefs based on religion instead of science.[385]

Once the belief in the superiority of plants for health was firmly entrenched in Western culture, most nutrition research became tainted by confirmation bias.[386] Confirmation bias is a term that describes a strong inclination to interpret research findings in a way that conforms to the researcher's existing beliefs.[387] The most notable example of this in nutrition research is Ancel Keys' Seven Countries Study. This study is still cited today as proof of the scientific evidence that eating saturated fat elevates blood cholesterol, "bad" LDL cholesterol, and leads to heart disease.[258] Although this so-called Diet-Heart Hypothesis has since been very convincingly proven wrong,[388,389] many people, including research scientists, are still influenced by the notion that restricting fat intake is required for optimal health. In actuality, a very large cohort study and other reviews of research have shown that high LDL cholesterol levels have very little value in predicting health risk.[390,391] In fact, over half the people who have heart attacks have normal LDL cholesterol levels.[391]

Additionally, there may be social pressures to adopt a more mainstream low-fat diet. Loved ones as well as complete strangers may feel it not only acceptable but necessary to instruct you on a proper diet. Authority figures in your life, such as respected family members or your medical provider, may admonish you to eat less fat. Despite her success in losing 35 pounds, decreasing her limb girth, resolving her pain, and increasing her energy and mental clarity, a patient of mine was cautioned by her doctor to stop eating ketogenically because her total cholesterol was elevated. Her physician insisted on treating the blood panel numbers rather than the person, his patient.

Because of all this history and undue influence, it now has become very difficult to find full-fat food options in a typical grocery store or restaurant. You are more likely to find a variety of low-fat, skim, or fat-free options than to find a product that contains more than a modicum of fat. A typical butcher's case is almost devoid of fat, leaving only very lean cuts of meat. A person must be especially assertive to let the butcher know that they desire the fat. This inability to understand that someone may actually want the fat that naturally comes with meat is not new. Arctic explorer Vilhjalmur Stefansson writes about his experience with trying to order a steak with the fat intact at a restaurant in the 1960 edition of his book *The Fat of the Land*. He describes giving up after the third attempt to communicate his desire to have the fat after each time being presented with a perfectly lean steak.[392]

Although we now know that consuming high levels of fat is safe and healthy, it remains unknown exactly how much fat is actually needed to best manage a lymphatic disorder. Results from animal studies have promising implications for people with lymphedema or other lymphatic disorders. Not only has a high-fat diet been shown as harmless to lymphatics,[249,250] it seems that dietary fat and ketones have tremendous potential for benefiting the lymphatic system.[28,29] Human studies are currently underway and will certainly add to what is known about nutrition in general and may also help us understand what is optimal for the lymphatic system.

Now that you are aware of potential pitfalls, misconceptions, and challenges you may face in adopting a ketogenic diet, you may feel better prepared to make the change. Or you may have already adopted this way of eating and now have a better understanding and can communicate your reasoning with greater clarity to others. Armed with that knowledge, you are now ready to move on to a discussion of the components of a healthy lifestyle beyond nutrition. In the next chapter, I will discuss what I believe you can do to not only improve the health of your lymphatic system, but optimize your health in general.

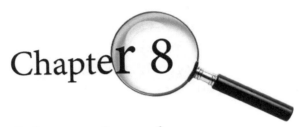

Chapter 8

Healthy Lifestyle ⇔ Healthy Lymphatics

"When once your point of view is changed, the very thing which was so damning becomes a clue to the truth."
—Sir Arthur Conan Doyle

I hope that I have successfully made the case in this book that a robust lymphatic system is vital to enjoying optimal health. This final chapter will put it all together by discussing the lifestyle choices that will promote lymphatic health.

All too often, the definition of healthy lifestyle is framed negatively by identifying habits which reduce your chances of serious illness or early death. This places the focus on what you should not do. I would rather place the emphasis on what you should do. What actions should you take to maximize the functioning of your lymphatic system, whether you have a lymphatic disorder or not? In this chapter, I discuss all of the essential aspects of lifestyle that are most beneficial to the lymphatic system, and thus to a healthy life. You will find that the components of a healthy lifestyle discussed in this chapter all influence and support each other. For instance, good nutrition provides energy that motivates you to exercise, improving sleep which in turn supports lymphatic clearance of debris in the brain.

Nutrition

Nutrition is the single most essential ingredient of a healthy lifestyle. In fact, I believe that without a consistently nutritious diet, optimal health can never be fully achieved. As I have described throughout this book, a deficient diet can severely impair the lymphatic system which has far reaching implications for your health. For this reason, I believe that a well-formulated ketogenic diet is key for a strong lymphatic system and good general health.

Improvements to your health through a proper diet can be seen in not only objective measures such as body composition and blood work, but also in more subjective assessments such as a feeling of improved energy and vitality, elevated mood, and enhanced clarity of thought. In a small pilot study of endurance athletes, after just ten weeks of a ketogenic diet they all reported a strong sense of general health and improved welfare.[393] I have witnessed this regularly in my own clinical practice and from a wide range of friends, family, colleagues and others with a lymphatic or fat disorder who have shared their experiences with dietary change. I suspect that the enhanced functioning of lymphatics in response to ketogenic eating has a profound role in this overall impression of well-being that is so universally reported.

One early noticeable effect of ketogenic eating is improved mental clarity. Concentration and the ability to focus and accomplish mental tasks are improved in many people within the first few weeks or months of adopting a ketogenic diet. The participants in two studies of healthy adults eating ketogenically noted enhanced mental focus and clarity, with one subject stating, "*I feel sharper mentally*".[393,394] It is not unusual to be unaware of the brain fog and poor concentration until it has lifted. One of my patients related how her improved clarity of thought allowed her to negotiate her way through a busy metropolitan airport, something she never would have considered she would be capable of before starting a ketogenic lifestyle.

> *"The best part for me was being able to accompany my granddaughter by plane, wait out the layover at the Phoenix Airport, deliver my granddaughter to our daughter and find my way back across the airport to my terminal. Such a major accomplishment for me!"* —Georgia S.

Another common outcome of eating ketogenically is a better disposition and fewer or less severe mood swings. A participant in one of the studies shared above stated that he was *"feeling very even in my moods (as in no real highs or lows)"*.[394] Improved emotional functioning with less negative emotion (such as depression, fearfulness, indecisiveness, moodiness and rage), less insomnia, and higher overall quality of life are reported in the literature.[395-397] It is not unusual to hear my patients report that they are much happier eating this way and see no reason to ever return to their previous diet.

Increased energy and vitality is a huge bonus of a ketogenic lifestyle. The boost of energy from this way of eating is especially evident once electrolytes are balanced and your body becomes more adept at using ketones and fat for energy rather than glucose. It is not uncommon to hear comments like *"I have heaps of energy"* and *"Feeling really good, energy levels are great!"*[394] One woman with lipedema reports this after just a few months of changing to a ketogenic diet:

> *"Let me start by saying just a few months ago I thought I was about two shakes from being in a wheelchair due [to] lipedema, but because of this way of eating this was my day: I swam for an hour this morning, went to Home Depot and was in there for about 2-1/2 hours on my feet, and I have been painting the rest of the day. Taking a small break, but have more to do. I can't believe I have been able to do all of this!!"* —K.S.M.

Certainly there is enhanced healing, growth and repair of skin, tissues, bones and muscle with ketogenic nutrition. Protein from animal sources especially makes for strong bones and healthy muscles[321,398] and ketosis stimulates wound healing and rebuilding of tissue.[399] Even more importantly, ketosis stimulates growth in the lymphatic system.[28,29] Although this miraculous property of ketones may be beneficial for anyone with a lymphatic system, the ability to generate new lymph vessels may prove to be monumentally pivotal in the life of someone living with a lymphatic disorder.

There is a large array of foods that are appropriate to a ketogenic lifestyle (see the Ketogenic Food List in Appendix I). Formulating a ketogenic eating plan that is most suited to you may require assistance from an expert who has knowledge of your health history and medical conditions as well as your food intolerances and preferences. Assembling a team that includes your lymphedema therapist, your doctor and other healthcare providers such as dietician or nutritionist that work in synergy and are supportive of your nutritional choices would be ideal, but not completely necessary. At least one expert who can monitor your health and offer advice on fine tuning your nutritional strategy will be satisfactory. See the Resources section for suggestions for finding health care professionals who may be able to help you.

Physical Activity and Exercise

Another vital part of a healthy lifestyle is physical activity and exercise. The physiological and psychological benefits of exercise are well-known and supported by both anecdotal reports as well as multiple research studies spanning the last century. Some of the noted benefits include improved cardiovascular health, increased muscle strength and bone density, improved balance and decreased risk of falls, improved breathing, reduced effects of stress, enhanced sleep, improved digestion, and elevated mood.

While the benefits of physical activity and exercise for general health are immense, they are no less so for the lymphatic system. In fact, movement and physical activity are vital factors in lymphatic function. For this reason, exercise is one of the essential components of Complete Decongestive Therapy, the gold standard for treatment of lymphedema and other lymphatic disorders.[400] The effectiveness of exercise for the management of lymphedema and lipedema has been demonstrated repeatedly in research, most often in the context of breast cancer treatment-related lymphedema.[401-404] Some experts have the opinion that exercise is so crucial to lymphatic health, it may even have an impact on preventing lymphedema in an at-risk population, or at least delaying the onset of it for many years.[405,406] I believe this may have been the case for Jean R. Because of her excellent level of fitness and daily physical activity, the onset of her cancer treatment-related lymphedema may have been delayed for more than twenty years:

> *"It all began with a hysterectomy for cervical cancer in my late twenties. The surgeon discovered cancerous nodes in my left groin and removed most of them. After the initial shock to my system (and almost dying), the swelling finally decreased, everything settled down and I was fine for twenty years.*
>
> *During that time, I was on my feet a lot teaching, chasing after two kids, running, skiing, biking, and the usual business of life, marriage, and career. Then suddenly in my late forties everything changed. I noticed that even though I elevated my swollen leg for hours, it would not go down."* —Jean R.

The muscle contraction associated with exercise is the primary mechanism to both encourage fluid in the tissues to be taken up by the initial lymphatics and to propel it along in the vessels once the lymph has successfully gained entrance. Contraction of muscles due to movement and exercise will result in decreased venous pressure, increased lymph flow, and increased muscle tissue pressure which all promote evacuation and transport of fluid.[406,407] Immobility, on the other hand, can have a tremendous negative impact on lymphatic function and can result in swelling and significant skin changes such as venous ulcers.[408] Secondary actions from exercise that improve lymphatic flow are the deeper breathing that accompanies exercise (discussed later in this chapter) and the repetitive movements which help soften tissue and reduce fibrosis.

Even with acknowledgement of incontrovertible evidence of the benefits of exercise, however, changing sedentary behavior can be just as challenging as changing diet. For one thing, you may suffer from other limiting health conditions and may even be in a great deal of chronic pain, which makes the prospect of exercise seem daunting.

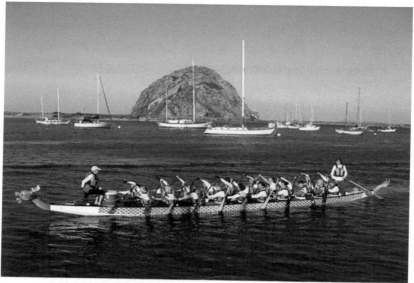

Figure 27. The author is steering the dragon boat for the Central Coast SurviveOars, a dragon boat team in Morro Bay, California made up of women who are cancer survivors. Many of the team members have lymphedema.

One of the primary benefits of a ketogenic lifestyle, as discussed above, seems to be reduction in fatigue and return of energy and vitality. Further, there is a great deal of evidence that a ketogenic diet can rapidly reduce pain which may increase interest in physical activity.[409,410] Lastly, burning fat for fuel reduces the production of lactate. Lactate is a metabolite that may contribute to pain during exercise and add to lymphatic load.[411] All of these factors may increase your desire for and pleasure in movement and physical activity. My recommendation is to engage in gentle movements to your tolerance until you begin to experience the decrease in pain and fatigue that comes with ketogenic eating. You will still make improvements and your lymphatic system will thank you by making you feel better. This plan of action is further supported by a 2017 study that showed that replacing a predominantly sedentary lifestyle with even light intensity movement/exercise for as little as six minutes every hour may be enough.[412] The important thing is just to move every day.

Although physical activity is important to optimal lymphatic functioning, exceeding your body's tolerance for exercise intensity may have a detrimental impact on lymphatic load and thus create more swelling. This is an especially important consideration if you have lymphatic impairment in your trunk. For this reason, experimentation, either on your own or with expert guidance, may be needed in order to determine what is right for you. I will provide you with some general guidelines for exercise here, but you may need to consult with a physical therapist, personal trainer, exercise physiologist or other professional who knows your medical history in order to develop your individual exercise plan.

The following section lists some general exercise guidelines found in the position statement on exercise developed by the Medical Advisory Board of the National Lymphedema Network (NLN). You can read more extensively on the NLN exercise recommendations by visiting https://lymphnet.org/position-papers.

1. Exercise is generally performed while wearing compression (such as compression bandages or garments).

2. Resistance exercises, such as lifting weights or using resistive bands, should be done with caution, starting with low weights, low repetitions, and gradual progression.

3. Allow adequate rest periods as needed

4. Maintain hydration.

5. Avoid exercising in extreme heat or getting overheated.

6. Regularly check the area of your body affected by lymphedema for symptoms (such as increased swelling or excessive fatigue compared to the rest of your body).

If you don't want to engage in an official exercise program, consider how you can incorporate short intervals of increased movement into your daily life. This can be done by parking further away from shops as you go about errands, walking the dog, or engaging in activities that require movement such as gardening or home repair projects. Taking the opportunity for movement throughout the day will benefit your lymphatic system the most. The following is a limited list of exercise suggestions. Of course, there are many more options of activities you may enjoy.

- Gentle Movement – chair yoga, Tai Chi, walking, water exercise.
- Graded Resistance – body weight resistance (push ups, sit ups), elastic bands, weights.
- Group and Individual sports – cycling, paddling, rowing, kayaking, Pickleball, tennis, badminton.

Perhaps the most effective, and consequently the most enjoyable, exercise that targets the lymphatics is movement that is performed in

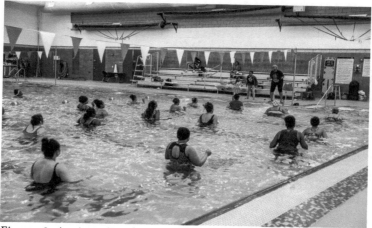

Figure 28. An Aqua Zumba class offered at Rainier Beach Community Center in Washington USA (Courtesy Seattle Parks and Recreation)

the water. This gentle, non-impact type of exercise is especially useful for someone who may be deconditioned, in pain, or have reduced mobility, as may be the case for someone with a lymphatic disorder. Additionally, if you are submerged to your chest or even to your neck, this means that almost your entire body is reaping the physiological effects of immersion in water. Although most research examining water exercise and lymphatic functioning has been performed with breast cancer survivors, there are a number of other studies that showed the benefits for lower body swelling and lipedema as well.[411,413,414] Study outcomes included reduced swelling, improved cardiovascular function, and reduced fatigue among other positive results.

The specific properties of water that make exercising while submerged more advantageous over land-based activities include: hydrostatic pressure, immersion diuresis, buoyancy, and viscosity. The effect of hydrostatic pressure creates a pressure gradient in which pressure increases with deeper immersion. If you are standing in the water, your feet are submerged the deepest and will have more compression. The compression gradually decreases toward the surface of the water. As much as 600 milliliters of fluid can be moved out of the legs if you are submerged to your chest.[415] This property of water means that compression garments are not necessary while exercising in the water. The fluid displacement from the legs up to the trunk due to hydrostatic pressure also has a direct impact on what scuba divers call *immersion diuresis*, or the increased urine production that occurs when a portion of our body is submerged under water. The need to urinate soon after exiting the pool is certainly satisfying to someone with fluid retention or a lymphatic disorder. This occurs due to the release of a hormone called *atrial natriuretic peptide*, or ANP, in response to the increased fluid volume moving to the heart. This hormone lowers blood pressure by stimulating the kidneys to release water.[416] Interestingly, ANP also increases ketone production, which we know helps with burning our body fat.[417]

Buoyancy is the tendency to float due to the support of the water pushing up against gravity. This property of water supports large heavy limbs and allows much greater pain-free range of motion than can ever be experienced on land. This may allow for better posture and improved gait and, most likely, decreased pain. Exercise can be more pleasurable when there is less weight-bearing and stress on joints. Further, if there is a gait disturbance due to large body size or asymmetry of limbs, exercise on land may contribute to further injury or damage. This can be avoided by instead moving in the water.

Water viscosity, or the thickness of water, allows us to grade exercise appropriate to each person. Using the resistance of water and its turbulence effects, you can make your exercise gentle or vigorous. The faster you move through the water, the more resistance you will feel, and thus can exercise harder if desired.[415] Water viscosity also has the ability to enhance the muscle-joint pump and facilitate lymph transport.[414]

There are some disadvantages to water exercise that may prove to be a barrier to participation. Social embarrassment due to poor body image can be an issue for some when donning a bathing suit and entering a public pool. Availability of a nearby pool and accommodations for disabled access may not be an option in your community. Finally, some medical conditions, the presence of an open wound, or incontinence would prevent pool use. Despite these potential barriers, many people find exercising in the water to be the best option for increasing their physical activity and managing a lymphatic disorder.

Breathing

Just as there are numerous benefits of physical activity and exercise, proper breathing can have a tremendous impact on all aspects of health. Breathing practices have been credited with lowering blood pressure, improving concentration, halting osteoporosis, and enhancing immune function. Slow deep breaths can help relieve stress and relax tense muscles. Controlled deep breathing can release endorphins that reduce pain. "Breathing is a missing pillar of health," claims James Nestor, author of the best selling book *Breath*.[418]

The power of breathing is even further entwined with lymphatic wellness. As discussed earlier in this book, breathing influences contraction of lymphatic vessels and improves lymphatic flow. Deep breathing with abdominal pressure applied by the therapist's hands has long been considered a vital component of complete decongestive therapy even while evidence for this practice is limited.[419] Lymphedema symptoms reduced more when deep breathing was incorporated into self-care practices in at least one study.[420] Moreover, the influence of breathing on optimal lymphatic performance may be most evident in the lungs themselves. Pulmonary lymphatics completely lack smooth muscle so are unable to use their own contractions to propel fluid. Yet they are able to absorb fluid more efficiently than blood vessels by relying predominantly on physiological properties of breathing.[168]

Although the impact of respiration on venous return has been rigorously studied, there is limited research investigating breathing and lymphatic function. It is well established that major blood vessels of the trunk are greatly influenced by contractions of the diaphragm as well as changes in pressure due to respiration, so it is logical to assume that the closely aligned lymphatic vessels are similarly

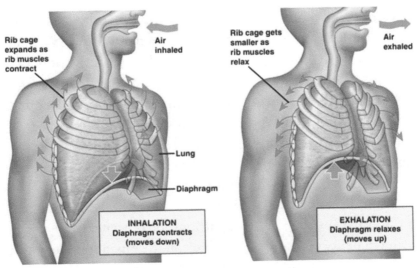

Figure 29. The action of the diaphragm with deep breathing

affected.[421] Deep diaphragmatic breathing is a powerful tool for management of lymphedema in the trunk and genitals especially. Even without lymphatic impairment in the trunk, activation of lymphatics in the body's core allows improved drainage from the limbs. And, as discussed in Chapter 1, deep breathing increases the contraction rate and lymph flow in the periphery and not just in the trunk.

According to Nestor, breathing deeply with a slow rate and through the nose creates a better balance of respiratory gases in our cells and promotes health. Nasal breathing improves sleep by reducing snoring, sleep apnea and fatigue.[422] Mechanically, the nasal passages are better equipped to filter out foreign particles and to humidify air than when breathing through the mouth. Most notable to lymphatic function, however, is the increased release of nitric oxide when you breathe through your nose rather than your mouth. This molecule has an impact on blood circulation, delivery of oxygen to cells, immune function and mood, but most important for the lymphatics, nitric oxide regulates lymphatic vessel contraction[423] and helps to maintain healthy lymphatic vessel walls.[45]

Gentle movement coordinated with breathing, as is used in yoga, Tai Chi and similar practices, seems to be very effective for enhancing lymphatic flow perhaps due to activation of the diaphragm. Kelly Bell has developed a breathing practice for the management of his truncal lymphedema and compromised lungs. He combines holding certain postures, breathing exercises, and abdominal pressure using his hand or a tool he has invented to enhance the effectiveness of his breathing. Kelly's protocol is described below, along with other breathing exercises.

Might breathing have an impact on overall lymphatic health over the entire life span, with or without the presence of a lymphatic disorder? I believe so, and encourage you to consider incorporating gentle exercise practices that stimulate deep breathing into your regular routine such as yoga or meditation. Described below are several breathing exercises that take only minutes and can be performed several times per day.

Kelly's Breathing Exercises – most beneficial for lymphedema in the trunk

1. Using a pillow under your hips and low back, position yourself as pictured below in Position 1. Your legs should be elevated with your knees bent and lower legs supported on a couch or chair. Cover yourself with a heated blanket to gently warm yourself.

2. Place your hand on your chest. Breathe in through your nose slowly as you tighten your core (abdomen). Your hand should feel your chest rising as you inhale.

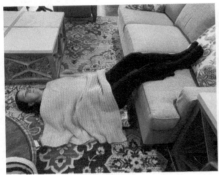
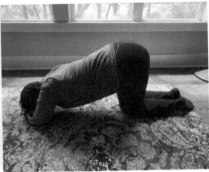

Position 1   *Position 2*

3. Every 5 minutes, over a period of 30 minutes, take 5 slow breaths.

4. Between each breath, tighten and lift your pelvic floor. (These are the muscles that you use to stop the flow of urine. You may have heard them described as Kegel exercises.)

5. Move into Position 2 pictured below, knees bent and resting your head on your forearms.

6. Repeat the breathing pattern described above by breathing in through your nose as you tighten your core over a period of 20 minutes.

7. Repeat pelvic floor contractions between breaths. If needed, you may repeat Position 1 for an additional 20 minutes.

Box or Square Breathing – increases focus and concentration

1. Sitting upright, exhale to a slow count of 4 through your mouth, getting all the oxygen out of your lungs.

2. Inhale slowly and deeply through your nose to a slow count of 4.

3. Hold your breath for another slow count of 4.

4. Exhale through your mouth for the same slow count of 4, expelling the air from your lungs.

Relaxing Breath (4-7-8 Breathing Technique) – increases relaxation with longer exhalation

1. Exhale completely through your mouth, making a whoosh sound.

2. Close your mouth and inhale quietly through your nose to a mental count of four.

3. Hold your breath for a count of seven.

4. Exhale completely through your mouth, making a whoosh sound to a count of eight. This is one breath.

5. Now inhale again and repeat the cycle three more times for a total of four breaths.

Sleep

One of the basic human physiological needs is sleep. Healthy sleep is such an essential function that it can impact every area of health and well-being including cognition, mood, energy, immune functions, hormonal balance, cardiovascular health and more. We spend a third of our life, more or less, engaging in sleep, and normally some part of every 24-hour day is devoted to this practice. This is a time for our body as well as our mind to relax, heal, and recharge, allowing us to wake refreshed and alert. It is no surprise, then, that optimizing your sleep is a necessary part of a healthy lifestyle.

The lymphatic system of our brain (glymphatics), as discussed in Chapter 4, does its best work while we sleep. The fluid space between brain cells becomes larger when we sleep, allowing the glymphatics free reign to clean up toxins and debris. Glymph flow increases by more than twofold during sleep, meaning a good night's rest may literally clear the mind.[189] It is interesting that everywhere else in the body, however, lymph flow slows down during sleep. Is that because blood pressure, heart rate, respiration, muscle contraction and sympathetic nerve activity are all slowed during sleep? Or is it because the sleeping posture is less gravity dependent? Some researchers believe that lymph flow in the body is reduced during sleep because lymphocytes (immune cells) are being retained in the lymph nodes where they can be most effective in destroying pathogens.[424] This is perhaps why we sleep more when we are ill: it allows much more time for a concentrated attack on noxious material in both our brain and our body.

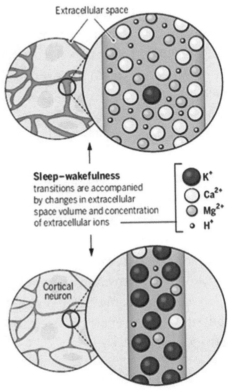

Figure 30. Brain shrinkage during sleep increases extracellular space and allows the glymphatics better access to clean up debris, toxins, and pathogens.

Deprivation or disrupted sleep patterns can lead to or exacerbate a host of chronic health problems. There are many circumstances that can interfere with sleep leaving us not only fatigued, but also less able to think clearly and make good decisions. This potentially leaves us vulnerable to a host of medical conditions. Disruption to sleep can be caused by pain, difficulty breathing, digestive upset (acid reflux, nausea), medication side effects, stress, or sleep rhythm disturbances (jet lag, rotating work shifts).

Wakening because of an urge to urinate is not unheard of for someone taking a diuretic (water pill), or because of a health condition such as a bladder infection. The most common reason for a nocturnal need to urinate, however, is because the hormone vasopressin, which directs your kidneys to hold water when you sleep, is ironically suppressed when you don't get enough sleep.[425] So poor sleep begets further poor sleep when you have to wake up, sometimes repeatedly, to urinate.

What can we do to improve our sleep? The best way is simply to follow practices that maximize sleepiness at bedtime. A well-formulated ketogenic eating plan may help. While a ketogenic diet had no impact on sleep for healthy individuals in one study,[426] sleep improved for healthy subjects in two others.[394,427] Sleep also improved for children with epilepsy and adults with obesity.[428-430] People with narcolepsy, a sleep disorder that causes overwhelming daytime drowsiness, report less sleepiness during the day while on a ketogenic diet.[431] This may be due to the blood sugar stabilization, and thus the improved energy level experienced with ketogenic eating, the opposite of which is encountered when eating a standard high carbohydrate diet.

Here are some more suggestions for slowing your mind and body down to prepare yourself for sleep, if you are having difficulty getting enough:

- Avoid exposure to electronics for at least 30 minutes before bed.
- Wear blue light blocking glasses after the sun goes down.
- De-stress in the evening: journaling, deep breathing exercises.
- Be physically active during the day.
- Avoid naps or sleeping in unless required for health reasons.
- Avoid large meals, caffeine, and alcohol within 2 hours of bedtime.

Other Sleep Promoting Measures

- Get out of bed when you can't stay asleep. Associate your bed with sleeping, not insomnia.

- Go to bed at the same time each night and get up at the same time each morning, including on the weekends. Being consistent will program your body to be sleepy at the right time.

- Make sure your bedroom is quiet, dark, relaxing, and at a comfortable temperature.

- Remove electronic devices, such as TVs, computers, and smartphones, from the bedroom.

Stress Management

Whenever we perceive that a challenge outweighs our ability to cope with it, we feel stress. Little and big stressors happen daily and are unavoidable. It may be a temporary annoyance such as being caught in traffic and worrying about being late for an appointment, or a longer term sort of trouble such as the stress of learning a new job or dealing with a debilitating illness. These two scenarios are examples of acute versus chronic stress. Chronic stress is generally viewed as being much more detrimental to our health, but both forms of stress can be harmful to our well-being depending on how we respond to a distressing situation. What really matters is how we keep it all at a manageable level. This is stress management.

It may be true that "reality is the leading cause of stress" as claims Rudy Boonstra, professor emeritus at the University of Toronto, in his 2012 paper with the same title.[463] He believes, from an ecology and evolutionary biology standpoint, even chronic stress in certain circumstances may prove to be adaptive and promote health. Although I don't necessarily subscribe to the maxim "What doesn't kill you, makes you stronger," I also don't believe that all stress is detrimental to health. At the same time, it is important to acknowledge that some aspects of life are genuinely stressful (often negatively) and outside of our ability to control. What we have some control over, however, is how we respond to various worries, fears, and concerns.

Dr. Jeremy Jamieson, at the University of Rochester's Department of Psychology, suggests that we reframe stressors as either challenges or threats. Although the sympathetic (fight or flight) nervous system is activated acutely in response to both challenging or threatening situations, a stressor redefined as a challenge may have a reduced physiological response. Using this model, negative stress can be changed to positive stress.[432] For instance, upon learning of their diagnosis of lymphedema, women who had survived breast cancer were initially very distressed and overwhelmed by the self-care demands necessary to manage their condition. Initially, the diagnosis of lymphedema was a threat, but after engagement in educational and supportive activities, they were able to reframe lymphedema as a challenge and were much more adherent to a self-care regimen.[433]

Our immediate response to stress is increased heart rate, blood pressure and breathing, and hormones such as cortisol and adrenaline are released. Immune functions are in a state of readiness and there is increased lymphatic flow.[434] Under conditions of chronic stress, however, this prolonged level of heightened arousal can be wearying and cause fatigue, irritability, sleep disturbance, impaired cognition, and suppressed immune functions.[435] Chronic stress can also lead to higher pain response, mood swings, and weight gain. There is lymphatic remodeling and decreased lymph flow with prolonged stress.[434,436]

Deep breathing and manual lymph drainage, two essential components of complete decongestive therapy for the treatment of lymphatic disorders, are both useful tools for reducing and managing stress. Quickened, shallow breathing and the constant increase in muscle tone associated with chronic stress impedes lymph flow and drainage. Conversely, slow deep breaths decrease autonomic nervous system (ANS) activity and feel very relaxing.[418] Manual lymph drainage, the specialized massage technique used to stimulate lymph flow to reduce swelling, was found to have a calming effect on the ANS in healthy people.[437] Perhaps this is why this technique is also beneficial for reducing pain, hypersensitivity, and anxiety.

Optimal nutrition will also support stress reduction and management. Although research on the effects of a ketogenic diet on psychological functioning and mental health has not been rigorous (studies have been small in size or only done in animal populations), anecdotal reports are certainly suggestive that good nutrition will support better management of stress.[438,439]

Other effective measures for managing stress include increasing your exposure to sunlight and enjoying nature, using relaxation techniques, engaging in consistent exercise or gentle movement activities, improving sleep, learning time management skills, and getting support from others. Fortunately, all of these practices happen to be strategies for optimizing the health of your lymphatics. The Mayo Clinic suggests four alliterative strategies for managing stress: avoid, alter, adapt and accept (See Figure 31.)

Stress Management Strategy 1: Avoid unnecessary stress	Stress Management Strategy 2: Alter the Situation
• Learn how to say "NO" • Avoid people who stress you out • Take control of your environment • Avoid arguments • Reduce your to-do list	• Express feelings calmly instead of bottling them up • Be willing to compromise • Be more assertive • Manage your time better

Stress Management Strategy 3: Adapt to the stressor	Stress Management Strategy 4: Accept the things you cannot change
• See your problems differently • Look at the big picture • Adjust your standards • Focus on the positive	• Don't try to control the uncontrollable • Look for the upside • Share your feelings • Learn to forgive

Figure 31. Practice the four A's of stress management (Mayo Clinic)

Sunlight

Being outside, especially on a warm sunny day, has a surprising influence on our well-being. Daily exposure to sunlight is important for our mood, bone growth, sleep quality, and immune function. It is unfortunate then, that we have spent the last four or five decades completely removing ourselves from the sun due to fear of skin cancer and premature aging. Although some caution is needed, I believe we have restricted our exposure to sunlight to such a degree that we are now vulnerable to depression, osteoporosis, sleep disturbances, and most relevant to the lymphatic system, infection. The benefits of sunlight are mostly related to three key hormones: vitamin D, serotonin, and melatonin.

Vitamin D is not considered an essential nutrient because we have the ability to make it ourselves, given enough exposure to sunlight. Sunlight, itself, should then be recognized as an essential nutrient. However, our ability to synthesize vitamin D in the skin in response to ultraviolet B (UVB) sunlight is often compromised.[440] Vitamin D, when supplied instead by diet, will be packaged into chylomicrons and then absorbed and transported by the lymphatic system. If produced in the skin in response to UVB rays, it travels in the blood using special vitamin D-binding proteins. Vitamin D is being studied for its potential influence in various mental health conditions including depression, seasonal affective disorder, schizophrenia, and autism.[441] There is a great deal of evidence that vitamin D deficiency is associated with increased risk and greater severity of infection, particularly of the respiratory tract.[442]

Serotonin acts as a hormone as well as a neurotransmitter. It allows brain and nerve cells to communicate with each other. Serotonin is of utmost importance for sleeping, eating, and digestion. Sunshine enhances serotonin levels in the body. There is a direct correlation between the amount of hours in bright sunlight and the rate of production of serotonin in the brain.[443,444] It is enlightening that morning sunlight may have the most beneficial effect on serotonin levels and mental health.[445] My friend and colleague Gail Straker follows the maxim of "sunlight before screen light," and enjoys the outdoors near her home in rural Idaho every morning before turning on her computer.

The third hormone of importance, melatonin, is of great importance for sleep. In fact, the more daylight exposure, the more melatonin you produce during the day. Levels will then go sharply up when the sun goes down, making you sleepy.[446] Melatonin has been found to reduce oxidative stress that can damage tissues, which may also have an impact on its role in reducing pain.[447,448] Recent studies have shown that melatonin may enhance the function of the immune system, of which the lymphatic system is an important part.[449] Getting plenty of exposure to sunshine during the day and keeping your bedroom dark at night will naturally increase your melatonin levels.

How much sunlight do you need to enhance your levels of these hormones? In general, at least five to fifteen minutes of sunlight, or longer if you are dark skinned, is recommended as the sweet spot between adequate yet not excessive enough to cause any health problems. Talk to your health care provider about what would be right for you and if you require supplementation.

Sunlight Exposure Considerations

- The season: In the winter, the sun is up for fewer hours and at a lower angle.
- The time of day: The sun's rays are most powerful between 10 a.m. and 3 p.m.
- Cloud cover/air pollution: The effects of the sun are diminished when it is occluded.
- Latitude: The sun is strongest and it is up longer year-round, closer to the equator.
- Skin Pigment: Higher melanin content darkens skin and requires more sun exposure to reap benefits.

Social Connections

Community and social connection is the glue that holds all of the other healthy lifestyle components together. Close relationships can have a huge impact on quality of life and physical and mental well-being. Connectedness to a community provides not only meaningful interaction and purpose, but a positivity and support that enhances overall quality of life as well.

There is significant evidence that a meaningful connection to others can lead to better weight and blood sugar management, improved cancer survival, decreased risk of death from cardiovascular disease, decreased symptoms of depression, and improved overall mental health.[450,451] Increasing your social connectedness by joining community groups, maintaining friendships and connections with family members, and participating in other social networks will not only add years to your life but may also improve the quality of those years.[451,452]

Commonality of meaning and purpose may be what draws you to particular people or groups in the first place. What motivates you or ignites your interest and passion? What do you want to be remembered for? Directing your energy toward those activities that are meaningful for you will have the most rewards. This is exemplified in one study in which women who identified themselves as "unemployed" felt more isolated than women who identified as "homemakers", even though both groups spent most of their time in the home.[453] I believe the difference may have been that the second group believed they were engaged in a meaningful activity, while the first group felt a loss of connection due to being unemployed. In the same study, those women who had more connection with their neighbors reported better mental outlook and health.

Positivity, or channeling your energy in a positive direction and away from the negative through your social interactions, is also an important factor. The health implications associated with more frequent positive emotions include fewer colds, reduced inflammation, and reduced risk of cardiovascular disease.[454-456] A group of researchers from the University of North Carolina in Chapel Hill hypothesized that there is a unique and powerful interaction between positive emotions, positive social connections and health outcomes.[457] Sixty-five university employees participated in their study, with half participating in a "loving kindness meditation practice" and the remainder in the control group. Results showed a significant impact on cardiac factors presumably from the positive emotions generated from the meditation practice. This led the researcher to speculate that *"positive emotions, positive social connections, and physical health influence one another in a self-sustaining upward-spiral dynamic."*[457]

Adopting a positive attitude can be challenging when coping with a chronic illness, however. Elizabeth McMahon, a clinical psychologist who has written extensively about the emotional challenges of lymphedema and lipedema, suggests that it is in your power to choose what to focus on. Although you are unable to change your diagnosis, you do have the power to change your habits, behaviors, expectations, as well as negative self-talk.[458]

As I will discuss in the next section about sustaining lifestyle change, developing meaningful social connections can support your ability to continue to make healthy lifestyle choices. Joining and actively engaging in groups that are aligned with your goals and beliefs can provide a sense of belonging, fulfill a need for friendships and social interaction, as well as furnish tangible emotional support. Investigate resources in your community for local options to make connections with like-minded people. Consider taking a community exercise or hobby class, attending a local special event that interests you, or joining a local special interest or activist group. See Resources (Appendix III) for suggestions for online support groups directed toward those with lymphatic and/or fat disorders and those interested in a ketogenic lifestyle.

Sustaining Lifestyle Change

Now that you have a clearer picture of the general lifestyle behaviors you want to change and why, how do you go about adopting these new habits? Within the range of behaviors that are healthy, how do you determine what is right for you? And how can you make a lasting change in your lifestyle that you feel is sustainable? In order to answer these questions, I will discuss how new habits are formed as well as some tips on sustaining those habits long term. Also examined here are different aspects of sustainability.

Habits are actions that we perform automatically without much thought, usually in response to some cue in our environment. For instance, we may have the habit of putting on a seatbelt in response to getting into a car. Although you may know what habits you want to adopt or change and why, it may still take some work to make your new health behaviors automatic. How do we translate an intention to change into actually enacting that change?

To increase your chances of being successful, the first step to developing a new habit should be to make a plan.[459] A good plan will include identifying the new behavior you want to adopt and the situations or conditions in which this new behavior will take place. For instance, if your new healthy behavior will be increasing your level of physical activity, the condition could be walking about your neighborhood at a set time each day. Your plan should include anticipating potential barriers to adopting the new behavior as well as how you will deal with those barriers. Knowing that excessive tiredness may keep you from walking, you may plan to implement your new habit earlier in the day before your fatigue becomes more severe. Start small and keep your expectations realistic. Continuing with the walking example, you might decide to walk only three times per week and just around one block, then, over time, increase the frequency and distance as you feel able. Good habits are worth the time and effort it takes to instill them.

Several factors contribute to making a new behavior automatic. The first is repetition. The more often you practice the new behavior, the more it becomes routine, and the greater chance there is for it to become habit.[460,461] Along with repetition, consistency is important. Doing your best to engage in the new behavior whenever the situation calls for it is an excellent practice and will increase the likelihood of habit formation.[461] Another factor is discovering the reward for your new behavior. Feeling less pain, more energy, and having less swelling can be very rewarding. Such positive benefits will tend to motivate you to continue to engage in your new habit. Additionally, performing your target behavior as part of your daily routine can help link it to environmental cues. For instance, donning your compression stockings can be cued by the act of getting out of bed, as this becomes part of your daily morning routine.

Another factor to consider in habit formation is that it is much more difficult to make a habit automatic if it is a complex behavior. For instance, it will be easier to adopt a new eating plan if you stick to a list of foods on your plan that you like to eat. Asking yourself, "Is this food on my list?" is much easier than having to consider whether each food will cause you harm or benefit before eating it. Take a look at the Ketogenic Food List in Appendix I and highlight those foods that you enjoy. This will then be your go-to list when developing the habit of eating a healthful ketogenic diet.

Sometimes, part of adopting a new habit is breaking an old habit that is, unfortunately, already ingrained. Breaking old habits can be aided by removing or changing environmental triggers that support those habits. Clearing out a pantry full of starchy foods effectively eliminates them as possible triggers. Becoming aware of what those patterns or triggers are for you is part of changing your habits. Make it easy to make good choices and to follow your plan. Be patient, as it takes time to implement changes and to realize the benefits. While you're waiting, imagine what your future will be like when you reap those benefits.

There are several aspects of lifestyle sustainability to consider, especially when deciding on adopting a new eating plan such as a ketogenic diet. The first aspect to consider is *can I sustain this way of eating for my lifetime?* This is really a question about managing long term adherence to your eating plan. It can be challenging to make any dietary change, but particularly to a way of eating that may not be completely supported by your family, friends, or medical providers. Steve D. shares his determination to get what he needed to support his new lifestyle from the hospital staff:

> *"The cafeteria at [the hospital I am in] is stuck in the 70s: lots of bread, potatoes, rice, sugar, and vegetable oils. I got in a shouting match with the cafeteria manager because they would send me margarine whenever I asked for butter. Luckily, my*

doctor was in favor of my trying a ketogenic way of eating, so he interceded on my behalf and I got my butter." —Steve D.

Social support, as discussed in the previous section, will be key to sustaining change. Encouragement from health coaches and online support groups, for instance, can be the reassurance you need to counteract any negative external pressures. Continue to educate yourself about lymphatic disorders and healthy lifestyle by listening to podcasts and attending conferences. Many educational opportunities are directed toward the layperson and are offered virtually and as in-person events. Please see Resources (Appendix III) for social networks and other sources for knowledge and support. For advice on your particular medical condition and the suitability of a ketogenic diet long term, find a medical provider that understands ketogenic nutrition in the Society of Metabolic Health Practitioners website listing.

One such opportunity for support in making lifestyle changes for people with a lymphatic disorder is offered by Robert Erkstam, an occupational therapist, life coach, and lymphedema therapist with a private practice in Wilmington, North Carolina. Robert offers my 12-week Lymphatic Lifestyle Solutions course to North Carolina residents and he modified it to be partly available online. Figure 32 provides

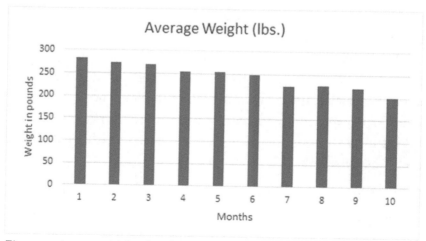

Figure 32: Average weight after the conclusion of the course is at Month 3. Average weight of participants continues to decline through Month 10.

some preliminary data from a group of his patients ten months after they graduated from his course. The data shows not just weight stabilization, but continued weight decline for participants as they continue to sustain lifestyle habit changes.

Other aspects of the sustainability of an eating plan that promotes consumption of animal-derived products has to do with environmental impacts, treatment of animals, financial feasibility, and the effect of the products produced on public health. Much of this is outside the purview of this book, but I will address these issues briefly. I would also direct the reader to the website, blog and "sodcast" of Dr. Peter Ballerstedt, a forage agronomist interested in a sustainable human diet through ruminant agriculture (See Resources).

Briefly stated, land populated by such ruminant animals as cows, sheep, and goats, is vastly superior for the environment than the millions of acres covered by monoculture crops. Consider that the mass production of plant foods such as wheat and corn requires the use of pesticides and herbicides whose purpose is to eliminate all life forms in the treated area that could potentially harm the crop. Meanwhile, the crops themselves leach so many nutrients from the soil that it must be left fallow every so often in a futile effort for the soil to heal and replenish its fertility. Most monocrop agriculture depends on unsustainable petrochemical fertilizers. Additionally, the diesel-energized heavy machinery used for harvesting kills millions of small animals, such as squirrels and lizards, during the reaping process. By contrast, cows roaming on a field improve the health of the soil by aerating it with their hooves and fertilizing it with their dung. It is not necessary to harm any insects or other animals to allow cows to forage, as all the life forms are behaving as part of a healthy ecosystem.

I would ask those who are concerned about the treatment of animals raised for the production of human food to consider all of the life forms that are maimed or completely annihilated in the process of crop production. If you are concerned for farm animal care and treatment, consider only purchasing beef that is grass-fed and finished to avoid supporting feedlots. Wild-caught fish and free-range chicken are also options. Support sustainable ranching and farming that consider welfare of animals and the environment in their food production. See Resources for links for more information.

Not least are other concerns of sustainability: economics and health. Can the producer be paid fairly for the product in order to conduct a profitable business? Can the workers be paid a fair wage? Lastly, health concerns override all other considerations. If a product results in harm to public health then it doesn't matter if the environment has been protected and the business is profitable to both the producer and the worker. This is the case with corn and soy. These crops are cheap to produce and can be transported around the world very economically, but they are responsible for most of humanity's chronic diseases. This is too high a cost. We need to rethink the advisability of a plant-based diet.

Thank you for reading my book.

My hope is that you have gained a better understanding of the lymphatic system, your health, and what constitutes a healthy lifestyle. With this new perspective, you can make more informed choices, experiment, learn, and continue to grow in ways that can improve your life and perhaps even have a beneficial impact on others. Thank you for joining me on this journey with Sherlock Holmes as we endeavored to crack

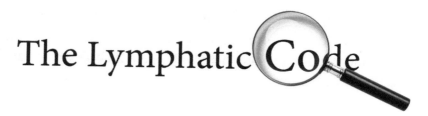

Appendices

". . . and meanwhile take my assurance that the clouds are lifting and that
I have every hope that the light of truth is breaking through."
—Arthur Conan Doyle, The Case-Book of Sherlock Holmes

Appendix I

Ketogenic Food List

As discussed in this book, ketogenic nutrition can be defined more by what is not eaten (carbohydrates) than by what you do consume. With that in mind, on the next page, you'll find a ketogenic shopping list. It contains examples of enjoyable items that can be included into a nourishing and delicious ketogenic way of eating. As you go through the list, highlight those foods that you enjoy. This will then be your go-to list when developing the habit of eating a healthful ketogenic diet. You'll notice that some of the vegetables have a star (*) by them. This denotes that they are relatively higher in carbohydrate, so you are advised to track consumption amounts carefully.

Bon Appètit!

Ketogenic Shopping List

Produce

- Leafy greens
- Artichokes
- Asparagus
- Broccoli
- Brussel Sprouts
- Cauliflower
- Celery
- Cucumber
- Eggplant
- Green Beans
- Jicama
- Leeks
- Mushrooms
- Okra
- Onions*
- Peppers*
- Squash*
- Tomatoes*
- Zucchini

Dairy Products

- Full Fat Cheeses
- Heavy Cream
- Sour Cream
- Cream Cheese
- Clotted Cream
- Creme Fraiche
- Turkish or Greek Yogurt

Meat and Other Proteins

- Bacon
- Beef
- Chicken
- Duck
- Eggs
- Fish
- Lamb
- Liver
- Organ Meats
- Pork
- Shellfish
- Turkey
- Veal
- Venison

Fats, Oils, Nuts and Seeds

- Avocado Oil
- Butter
- Coconut Oil
- Ghee
- Lard
- Mayonnaise
- Olive Oil
- Almonds
- Brazil Nuts
- Macadamia Nuts
- Pecans
- Pumpkin Seeds
- Sunflower Seeds
- Walnuts

Beverages

- Water
- Carbonated Unsweetened Flavored Water
- Coffee
- Tea

Appendix II

Glossary of Terms

Adaptive immunity	A targeted but slower immune response to pathogens.
Adipocytes	Fat cells (cells which store fat in the body)
Adipose	Connective body tissue composed mostly of adipocytes.
Anchoring filaments	Specialized filaments that prevent lymphatic capillaries from collapsing.
AND	Academy of Nutrition and Dietetics
ANP	Atrial Natriuretic Peptide
Antigens	Toxins, bacteria, viruses and other foreign invaders.
Arterial capillary	The tiniest blood vessel that transports nourishment to cells.
CDT	Complete Decongestive Therapy.
CEUS	Contrast-Enhanced Ultrasound. Imaging that uses a contrast agent along with sound waves to visualize lymph nodes and vessels.

CHF	Congestive Heart Failure. A chronic condition of the heart.
Chyle	The milky white lymphatic fluid found in the abdominal lymphatics.
Chylous ascites	A malady involving an accumulation of lipid-rich lymph that has leaked into the abdominal cavity.
CICO	Calories in, Calories Out. A theory of energy balance.
Cisterna chyli	An enlarged sac that constitutes the beginning of the thoracic duct.
Congenital lymphedema	Lymphedema that appears at birth.
Continuous blood vessel	The most common form of a blood capillary that only allows very small particles and fluid to exit.
COPD	Chronic Obstructive Pulmonary Disease. A group of lung diseases.
CVI	Chronic Venous Insufficiency. A condition in which leg veins become unable to transport blood adequately.
Dendritic cells	Specialized white blood cells that patrol the body for pathogens, which are then delivered to the lymph nodes.
Diuretics	Water pills.
DVT	Deep Vein Thrombosis, also known as a blood clot.
Fat adaptation	Also, Fat-adapted. The body has successfully converted to efficiently metabolizing fat for fuel rather than carbohydrates.
Fenestrated blood vessel	A blood capillary with intermediate-sized openings that allow the exit of fluid and particles.

Filariasis	A parasitic infection that causes harm to the lymphatic system, resulting in lymphedema.
Forward cholesterol transport	The process of bringing cholesterol to the tissues from the liver.
Gluconeogenesis	The conversion by the body of proteins and triglycerides into glucose.
Glycocalyx	A gel-like carpet made up of tiny hair-like extensions that cover and protect the lining of blood and lymph vessels.
Glymphatics	Specialized lymphatics of the central nervous system (brain and spinal cord).
HCG	Human Chorionic Gonadotropin.
HDL	High Density Lipoprotein.
Hemosiderin staining	A dark brown stain on the lower calves, often due to CVI.
Hyper –	High or higher.
Hyperglycemia	High blood sugar.
Hypo –	Low or lower.
Hypoglycemia	Low blood sugar.
Immersion diuresis	The increased urine production that occurs when a portion of the body is submerged under water.
Immune tolerance	The variable amount of toxin that can be tolerated by the human immune system.
Inguinal nodes	Lymph nodes found at the groin.
Innate immunity	The inborn natural defense that is broad and non-specific, but rapid.

ICG	Indocyanine Green. A diagnostic dye that allows for real time visualization of the contraction of lymph vessels and location of lymph nodes.
Insulin resistance	A reduced response to the hormone insulin.
Interstitial fluid	Fluid and particles in the tissues, before they enter the lymphatic system.
Interstitial space	The space between cells in the body's tissues.
Ketogenic diet	A way of eating that promotes ketone production. Also referred to as keto or low carbohydrate in this book.
Ketones	Fatty acid metabolites that can be used as an efficient energy source.
Ketosis	Metabolic process of utilizing fat as an cellular energy source.
Lacteal	Lymph capillaries found in the intestine that absorb dietary fat.
LCHF	Low Carb, High Fat.
LDL	Low Density Lipoprotein.
Lipo-lymphedema	The diagnosis when both lipedema and lymphedema occur together.
LPL	Lipoprotein Lipase.
Lumbar trunk	A large lymphatic vessel that travels from the groin to the deep pelvic nodes in the trunk.
Lymph	A colorless fluid containing white blood cells, proteins, water, waste products and fat.
Lymph heart	Little propulsion structures that pump lymph in amphibians, reptiles and flightless birds.
Lymph sacs	Embryonic beginnings of lymph vessels.

Lymphangiogenesis	Lymph vessel generation.
Lymphangiography	Also called lymphography, an imaging technique for the lymphatic system.
Lymphangion	The segment between valves in a lymphatic vessel that contract to pump lymph.
Lymphangio-scintigraphy	Also called lymphoscintigraphy, lymphatic imaging that uses a radioactive tracer.
Lymphatic vasa vasorum	Lymphatic vessels that drain larger arteries.
Lymphedema Praecox	Lymphedema that appears before age 35.
Lymphedema Tardum	Lymphedema that appears after age 35.
Lymphocytes	Immune cells that are trained to recognize certain foreign matter and build an immune response.
Macrophages	Immune cells that engulf and eliminate any invaders.
MCT	Medium Chain Triglyceride.
Mesenchymal cells	Primitive cells that are able to develop into connective tissue, blood vessels, or lymphatic vessels, depending on need.
Metabolism	The sum of all catabolism and anabolism going on in the body.
MI	Myocardial infarction. Also known as heart attack.
Myelin sheath	An insulating layer of fat surrounding nerves that facilitates electrical impulses.
NSV	Non-Scale Victory.
Nutritional Ketosis	When ketone levels in the blood reach at least 0.5 millimolars per deciliter due to a healthy dietary intake.
PCOS	Polycystic Ovary Syndrome.

Peyer's patches	Lymph node-like organs in the lining of the small intestine that test food for toxins and initiate an immune response.
PF4	Platelet Factor 4. A possible biomarker for lymphatic dysfunction.
Phlebo-lymphedema	The coexistence of venous and lymphatic disease.
Popliteal nodes	Lymph nodes found behind the knee.
Protein-losing enteropathy	Damage to the intestinal lining which causes excessive loss of protein.
Reactive fibrosis	Fibrosis that occurs in the tissues in response to inflammation due to lymphedema.
Reverse cholesterol transport	Delivery of excess tissue cholesterol through the lymphatic system back to the liver.
Right lymphatic duct	A large lymphatic vessel that drains the right side of the trunk, right arm and right side of the head and neck.
RNY	Roux-en-Y bariatric surgery.
RQ	Respiratory Quotient.
SAD	Standard American Diet.
Sentinel lymph node biopsy	A small sampling of lymph nodes to test for cancer.
Sinusoid blood vessel	The leakiest of the blood vessels that allow large particles and fluid to exit.
Stemmer sign	The inability to lift the skin at the base of the toes or fingers
Thoracic duct	The largest lymphatic vessel in the body, located in the trunk.
T-lymphocyte cells	Immune cells that develop from stem cells in the bone marrow and the thymus gland.

Triglyceride	Three fatty acid molecules attached to a glycerol molecule.
Vasa vasorum	Highly permeable blood vessels that feed larger arteries.
Venous Reflux	Venous blood flows back into the tissues.

Appendix III

Resources

Lymphatic Education

- Leslyn Keith, OTD, CLT-LANA (http://leslynkeith.com)
- Klose Training & Training (https://klosetraining.com)
- Lymphatic Education & Research Network (https://lymphaticnetwork.org)
- The Lipedema Project (https://lipedemaproject.org)
- Lipedema Simplified (http://lipedema-simplified.org/keto)
- National Lymphedema Network (https://lymphnet.org)
- Allyson's Story (growing up with primary lymphedema) Klose Training Videos

Diet & Health Websites

- Central Coast Nutrition Conference (http://www.ccnutritionconference.com)
- Dr. William Davis, Wheat Belly (https://www.wheatbellyblog.com)

- Dr. Andreas Eenfeldt, Diet Doctor
  (https://www.dietdoctor.com)
- Dave Feldman, Cholesterol Code (https://cholesterolcode.com)
- Ellen Davis, Ketogenic Diet Resource
  (https://www.ketogenic-diet-resource.com)
- Ivor Cummins, The Fat Emperor
  (https://thefatemperor.com/blog)
- Lipedema and Keto: (https://keto.lipedema-simplified.org/)
- Low Carb USA (http://www.lowcarbusa.org)
- Low Carb Down Under (http://lowcarbdownunder.com.au)
- Low Carb Action Network (https://lowcarbaction.org/)
- Public Health Collaboration UK (https://phcuk.org)
- Kidney Stones (https://kidneystones.uchicago.edu/)
- Dr. Ben Bikman's company (https://www.insuliniq.com/)
- Grassroots Health Nutrient Research Institute (https://www.grassrootshealth.net/)
- Own Your Labs Blood Testing Services
  (https://ownyourlabs.com/)

Educational Opportunities

- Lipedema Simplified MasterClass program
  (https://lipedema-simplified.org/masterclass-program-2021/)
- Carnivore Con (https://carnivorycon.com/)
- Low Carb Denver conferences
  (https://lowcarbconferences.com/)
- Ketogenic Solution for Lymphatic/Fat Disorders Symposia
  (https://lipedema-simplified.org/ketogenic-solution-for-lipedema-lymphedema-mini-symposium-2021/)

- Low Carb USA conferences (https://www.lowcarbusa.org/)
- Proper Human Diet Summits (https://drberry.com/proper-human-diet/)
- Noakes Foundation Nutrition Network (https://nutrition-network.org/)
- Dr. Eric Westman - Adapt Your Life Academy (https://adaptyourlifeacademy.com/)

Food Log Websites

- Carb Manager (https://www.carbmanager.com/)
- Cronometer (https://cronometer.com/)
- KetoDiet (https://ketodietapp.com/)
- MyFitnessPal (https://www.myfitnesspal.com/)
- Total Keto Diet (https://www.totalketodiet.com/)

Low-Carb Healthcare Providers

- Jeffry Gerber (https://denversdietdoctor.com)
- Jeff Volek, Steve Phinney & Sarah Hallberg Virta Health (https://www.virtahealth.com)
- Franziska Spritzler (http://www.lowcarbdietitian.com)
- Society of Metabolic Health Practitioners (https://thesmhp.org/)
- Dr. Eric Westman, Duke Keto Medicine Clinic (https://medicine.duke.edu/faculty/eric-charles-westman-md)
- Dr. Jay Wortman, Vancouver, BC, Canada (https://www.docsonthebay.ca/physicians)

Videos On YouTube:

- Leslyn Keith YouTube Channel (https://www.youtube.com/channel/UC4g7g72sTTHZQso-JFnLdSg)
- Kelly Bell interview (https://www.youtube.com/watch?v=LUqMNpCc3sw)
- Dr. Jay Wortman, My Big Fat Diet (https://www.youtube.com/watch?v=GxAztFu6ugA)
- Dr. Thomas Seyfried, Cancer as a Metabolic Disease (https://www.youtube.com/watch?v=SEE-0U8_NSU)
- Dr. Jeff Volek, The Many Facets of Keto-Adaptation (https://www.youtube.com/watch?v=n8BY4fyLvZc)
- Prof. Ken Sikaris, Cholesterol, When to Worry (https://www.youtube.com/watch?v=OyzPEii-wo0)
- Cereal Killers Movie (https://www.dietdoctor.com/watch-the-lchf-movie-cereal-killers-for-free)
- Dr. Ted Naiman, Insulin Resistance (https://www.youtube.com/watch?v=Jd8QFD5Ht18)
- Dr. Robert Cywes, Diabetes Understood (https://www.lowcarbusa.org/videos/diabetes-understood-series/)
- Tom Naughton: Fat Head (https://www.fathead-movie.com)
- Shawn Baker, MD (https://www.youtube.com/channel/UC5apkKkeZQXRSDbqSalG8CQ)

Videos on the Lymphatic Education & Research Network:

- Diet and Lifestyle for Lymphatic Disorders: Implementing a Ketogenic Diet (https://lymphaticnetwork.org/symposium-series/presenters/leslyn-keith)

- The Science and Practice of Low Carb/High Fat/Ketogenic Way of Eating for Lymphatic Disorders (https://lymphaticnetwork.org/symposium-series/presenters/Dr.-eric-westman)

Social Media – Facebook Groups

- Keto and Fasting for Lymphedema (https://www.facebook.com/groups/342880423166729)
- Keto Lifestyle for Lipedema (https://www.facebook.com/groups/LipedemaKetoWOE/)
- Low Carb Support Group By Dr. Eric Westman (https://www.facebook.com/groups/DukeLowCarbSupportGroup/permalink/1929388043806637/)

Books

- Baker, S. *The Carnivore Diet.* Las Vegas, NV: Victory Belt Publishing. 2020.
- Bikman, B. *Why We Get Sick.* Dallas, Texas: BenBella Books. 2020
- Christofferson T. *Tripping Over the Truth.* Hartford: Chelsea Green Publishing, 2017.
- Cummins I, Gerber J. *Eat Rich, Live Long.* Las Vegas, NV: Victory Belt Publishing. 2018.
- Davis E. *Fight Cancer with a Ketogenic Diet.* Cheyenne: Gutsy Badger Publishing, 2013.
- Davis E, Runyan K. *The Ketogenic Diet for Type 1 Diabetes.* Cheyenne: Gutsy Badger Publishing, 2014.
- Davis E, Runyan K. *Conquer Type 2 Diabetes with a Ketogenic Diet.* Cheyenne: Gutsy Badger Publishing, 2014.
- Davis W. *Wheat Belly: Lose the Wheat, Lose the Weight, and Find Your Path Back to Health.* Rodale Books, 2014.

- Davis W. *Wheat Belly Cookbook: 150 Recipes to Help You Lose the Wheat, Lose the Weight, and Find Your Path Back to Health.* Rodale Books, 2012.

- DiNicolantonio, J. *The Salt Fix.* New York, New York: Harmony Books. 2017.

- Feinman RD. *The World Turned Upside Down.* Brooklyn, New York: NMS Press; 2014.

- Gedgaudas NT. *Primal Body, Primal Mind, Beyond the Paleo Diet for Total Health and a Longer Life.* Healing Arts Press; 2011

- Kraft JR, Fcap JR. *Diabetes Epidemic & You.* Trafford on Demand Pub, 2008.

- Keith, Lierre, *The Vegetarian Myth: Food, Justice, and Sustainability.* Crescent City, California: Flashpoint Press. 2009

- Kwaśniewski J. *Homo Optimus.* Warsaw, Poland: WGP Publishing. 2000.

- Masino SA (Ed.) *Ketogenic Diet and Metabolic Therapies: Expanded Roles in Health and Disease.* New York, New York: Oxford University Press. 2016.

- Monastyrsky, K. *Fiber Menace*, Ageless Press, 2005

- Moore J, Westman EC. *Cholesterol Clarity.* Victory Belt Publishing, 2013.

- Naiman, T., Shewfelt, W. *The P:E Diet: Leverage your biology to achieve optimal health.*

- Noakes, T, Sboros, M. *The Eat Right Revolution: Your Guide to Living a Longer, Healthier Life.* Cape Town, South Africa: Penguin Random House. 2021.

- Perlmutter D, Loberg K. *Grain Brain.* New York, NY: Little, Brown and Co., 2013.

- Rodgers, D, Wolf, R. *Sacred Cow: The Case for (Better) Meat.* Dallas, Texas: BenBella Books. 2020.

- Simmonds A. *Principia Ketogenica, Compendium of Science Literature on the Benefits of Low Carbohydrate and Ketogenic Diets.* Createspace; 2014.

- Stefansson, V. *The Fat of the Land.* (Originally: *Not By Bread Alone*, MacMillan Company, 1960)

- Teicholz N. *The Big Fat Surprise: Why Butter, Meat and Cheese Belong in a Healthy Diet.* New York, New York: Simon & Schuster, 2015.

- Taubes G. *Good Calories, Bad Calories: Fats, Carbs, and the Controversial Science of Diet and Health.* New York: Anchor Books, 2008.

- Taubes G. *Why We Get Fat, and What to Do About It.* New York: Anchor Books, 2011.

- Taubes, G. *The Case for Keto.* New York, New York: Alfred A. Knopf. 2020.

- Volek JS, Phinney SD. *The Art and Science of Low Carbohydrate Performance: A Revolutionary Program to Extend Your Physical and Mental Performance Envelope.* Boca Raton: Beyond Obesity LLC, 2012.

- Westman E, Berger, A. *End Your Carb Confusion: A Simple Guide to Customize Your Carb Intake for Optimal Health.* Victory Belt Publishing, 2020.

Carnivore Diet and Sustainable Ranching

- Carnivorous way of eating: (https://www.carniway.nyc/) and his page about plant toxins (Planti-nutrients) (https://www.carniway.nyc/plantinutrients)

- Meat Rx (https://meatrx.com/)

- Peter Ballerstedt Blog and Sodcast (http://grassbasedhealth.blogspot.com/)

- Adventures in Diet by Arctic Explorer Vilhjalmur Stefansson (initially published by Harper's Monthly Magazine, November 1935) (http://www.comby.org/documents/documents_in_english/stefansson-diet-adventures.htm)

- Amber O'Hearn website, online book and blog: Eat Meat. Not too Little. Mostly Fat. (https://www.mostly-fat.com/)

Appendix IV

Making Keto Fit Your Budget

It is likely that you will find that a ketogenic way of eating is generally less expensive than your previous diet. If your diet used to be relatively omnivorous, you were likely already buying meats, eggs, dairy and fresh vegetables. Now you are actually buying less because you aren't also purchasing bread, pasta, cereals, and other highly packaged/processed foods. While before, an 8-ounce steak would only last for one meal, now it lasts for three because you eat all of the fat that comes with it and it fills you up more. By eliminating the starchy foods from your meal, you feel satiated with less food. You stay satiated longer, which does away with the need for snacking two hours after a meal. You certainly can spend more by always purchasing organic, free-range, wild-caught, and grass-fed options, but you don't have to. Even the cheapest eggs, poultry, fish and beef will still be healthier than a high carbohydrate diet. Purchase those more expensive options as you are able to afford it.

But you don't just save on your grocery bill. You also require fewer supplements. By focusing on eating real foods, you increase the likelihood you will be getting all of the essential nutrients, vitamins, and minerals from foods instead of pills. As your health improves, your health care costs go down with decreased medications, fewer co-pays, lower insurance premiums, and reduced risk for costly hospitalizations. Chronic conditions like diabetes and heart disease can severely strain your budget, not to mention your quality of life. All the money you save on healthcare costs can be used instead for things that give you pleasure: a visit to a spa, a new car, a trip to visit friends or relatives you haven't seen in a long time.

Additional Tips for Keto on a Budget

- Stock your freezer with things that can be purchased on sale and frozen

- Cook at home (a home cooked meal offers you more control over ingredients, tastes better, and is less costly than restaurant eating)

- When you do eat out, ask about the a la carte menu so you don't have to pay for unwanted starchy side dishes.

- When you have friends over, don't feel you have to incur the expense of catering to their dietary choices. (Stick to your plan. Most people find keto food delicious and won't miss bread or baked potatoes.)

- Buy a roast (which is generally much cheaper than steak) and slice it/cook it like steaks.

- Ground meat, pork and chicken are less expensive options compared to beef.

- Check store circulars and buy what is on sale, whatever that keto food might be. My Grocery Deals (https://www.mygrocerydeals.com/) is a grocery discount aggregator.

- Search the web or YouTube for "keto on a budget" for more great ideas.

Appendix V

Personal Stories

Georgia S.

Yes, I have lipedema, diagnosed stage 2 and I am 73. Three and a half years ago, as I sat in my doctor's office with my breathing problems (asthma since age 3), I met a former acquaintance. This lady phoned Dr. Keith, a mutual acquaintance, with concerns of how ill I looked. Soon I was speaking with Dr. Keith, having my legs measured and beginning a keto way of eating. My legs were so swollen and the pain was uncomfortable! I was using a cane or walker with the realization that a wheelchair was my future.

I have been keto now for three and a half years with a loss of 46 pounds. My legs are much smaller and the pain has diminished. I think clearer and my energy level is better than it was 20 years ago. Since I am healthier, I have found that I don't seem to catch colds or become ill as often as I used to, which has also helped with my asthma. The best part for me was being able to accompany my granddaughter by plane, wait out the layover at the Phoenix Airport, deliver my granddaughter to our daughter and find my way back across the airport to my terminal. Such a major accomplishment for me!

The past 8 months I have eaten mostly Carnivore and continue to feel fairly well despite having another major surgery at the end of last year and then catching an illness just a few months ago. This illness placed me on four breathing meds for two months. I eat one to two times a day during a 6-8 hour time period. My fasting is usually between 16-20 hours because I just do not get hungry. I also do not obsess about my weight and only check it monthly. I believe I gained a couple pounds back due to the hip surgery and lung issues. Sometimes, in the past couple months, a warm piece of pie seemed to wrap its arms around me – a comfort food, I guess. I do find that if I go off-plan with my eating I definitely do not feel as good. This experience makes it easy for one to jump right back into keto.

Additionally, I do the self-care techniques of self-drainage, dry brushing, moisturizing my legs, vibration plate for 10-20 minutes, compression garments, pumping my legs for an hour a day and epsom salt baths. Generally, I perform most of the self-care daily depending upon my stamina in order to remain as ambulatory as I can. My love is being outside in my garden for 2-3 hours a day, which gives me exercise and vitamin D.

Lipedema, as with any disease, has its challenges and is difficult on our physical, mental and emotional well-being! Don't let your body define who you are as you are sooo much more! "Special You" are your heart, soul and mind. You are loved by many. I try to remind myself that taking care of myself is the best gift I can give to myself, my husband, adult children and all those I love. YOU CAN DO THIS, we Lippies are STRONG!

DATE	1/18/2017	7/23/2019
Weight	232.3	194.4
Total Body Water	91.2	86.6
Body Fat (lbs)	93.6	74.2
B.M.I	36.4	30.5
% Body Fat	42.5	38.2

Other stats (after 18 months on keto):

- Total Leg Volume Decrease – right leg = 2872.6 ml
  left leg = 2959.0 ml
- Bilateral Extracranial Arterial Duplex – Unremarkable
- Coronary Artery Calcium Score – 0

Georgia S.

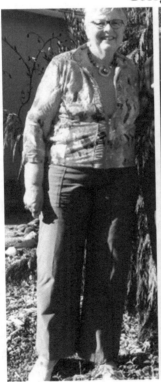 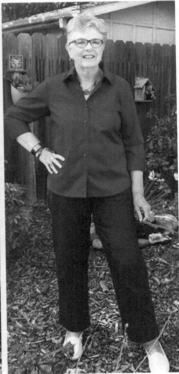

Two months after starting diet   *Eighteen months after starting diet*

Steve D.

I have a memory of looking down at my leg after a blunt object had been pressing up against it and seeing a deep pit. I can't remember how old I was, where I was, or what the blunt object was, but I remember thinking it was cool! I also recall playing in rock 'n roll bands in my mid-twenties and my legs feeling heavy when I climbed the steps to the stage. Then, one hot and humid day when I was in my thirties, I mowed a very large yard. Later that night, I awoke from my sleep with a searing pain in my left leg. It was cellulitis, the first time of dozens, if not hundreds, that were to come. Within a few months of that first bout, my left leg was twice its former size. I had also put on a lot of "weight." I was standing in line somewhere and felt like my legs wouldn't hold me much longer. I went to see a doctor. He walked in, took one look at me, and told me I was too fat and that was causing my leg to swell. Shortest doctor's appointment ever.

Fast forward to Y2K: I moved to another city and within days of arriving here, I went to the ER with cellulitis. I was prescribed antibiotics, by now a familiar ritual. On my way out, I glanced down at the receipt I had been given. The words "morbid obesity" caught my eye. About a year later, I hit my right leg hard against the corner of the metal frame of my bed and developed what turned out to be a chronic wound that took a long time to heal.

About a year prior to this time, I started the Zone diet, all the rage back then. After two years, I'd lost 135 pounds and felt like I had my life back, although the cellulitis episodes continued. Then I hit a weight loss plateau that was more like The Great Plains. I was also starving, because the Zone diet, despite its fancy scientific jargon, is basically a very low calorie diet. I went off the diet and the weight just poured back on. I was so hungry, I couldn't stop eating. I started getting cellulitis on my thighs, my torso, and my belly and developing skin changes. By this time, I had been to the hospital (which I will call VMC) countless times for cellulitis. Not a single doctor or nurse ever said one word about the horrible skin on my belly, so again, I assumed it was due to my obesity.

In 2012, I went back to VMC with a bad case of cellulitis. My extended stay without getting out of bed led to six months in two different nursing homes. I eventually was walking again, but at nowhere near the same level of ability as before. After I got back home, a home health care nurse came to check on me. She took one look at my swelling and bumpy skin and said "You have Stage 3, advanced lymphedema and that rough skin is called 'induration.'" Finally, after twenty-some years, I was diagnosed! I went online and did some research and sure enough, the symptoms described me to a "T." I also learned that Stage 3 lymphedema is irreversible.

In 2014, I found myself back at VMC with cellulitis. I insisted they get me out of bed every day, but the physical therapist refused! I couldn't understand what was going on. It never occurred to me to tell them I could walk, any more than I would think to tell them I could see. I later realized that they must have simply assumed I couldn't walk due to my size. I wound up unable to walk again and in another nursing home, but this time the nursing home failed to provide me with the level of physical therapy I needed to get back on my feet. At this point, I was declared a permanent nursing home resident, incapable of rehabilitation.

After fourteen months in this nursing home, I developed a fever of 103 degrees F and had to come back to VMC; this was in July of 2015. Once I was better, they tried to force me to return to the nursing home, but I refused. After six months of not getting out of bed, out of desperation, I posted a video online asking for help. My sister had the brilliant idea of posting my video in several Lymphedema groups on Facebook. A total stranger reached out to her and told her he could help me. This stranger turned out to be my hero, Mr. Kelly Bell. He told me his own harrowing tale of lymphedema and how he got his life back thanks to the ketogenic diet.

The cafeteria at VMC is stuck in the 70s: lots of bread, potatoes, rice, sugar, and vegetable oils. I got in a shouting match with the cafeteria manager because they would send me margarine whenever I asked for butter. Luckily, my doctor was in favor of my trying a ketogenic way of eating, so he interceded on my behalf and I got my butter. I was able to do what I call "hospital keto," which is the closest I could get to a true ketogenic diet, given my choices here. It worked! I lost 100 pounds in a year. Added to the 50 pounds I had managed to very slowly lose just by making wiser food choices, I'm down 150 pounds My legs look normal for the first time in years. I still carry a lot of lymph fluid on the left side of my torso and my belly, but much less than before. I haven't had cellulitis again in ages and my skin is in much better condition. I'll always be grateful to Kelly for the information and support he's given me. I was inspired to help others, as he had helped me. I started a Facebook group called "Keto and Fasting for Lymphedema." We're closing in on 1,600 members.

Believe it or not, I'm still at VMC six years later, still not walking. I would have to write a whole book to explain how that can be, but at least now they've assigned a therapist to work with me every day, so I'm getting some pretty intense workouts in bed. I have way more energy, but it is hard to compare to before when I was walking. I do know I'm luckier than countless others with lymphedema who are not getting help, perhaps because their medical providers don't even know what lymphedema is. I know I WILL walk again!

Jean R.

My Journey With Lymphedema

If you graphed my journey with lymphedema, it would look like the stock market: up, down, sometimes flat. It all began with a hysterectomy for cervical cancer in my late 20s. The surgeon discovered cancerous nodes in my left groin and removed most of them. After the initial shock to my system (and almost dying), the swelling finally decreased, everything settled down and I was fine for twenty years.

During that time, I was on my feet a lot teaching, chasing after two kids, running, skiing, biking, and the usual business of life, marriage, and career. Then suddenly in my late 40s everything changed. I noticed that even though I elevated my swollen leg for hours, it would not go down. After consulting with a nurse practitioner, she informed me that I had a condition called "lymphedema." No one had ever mentioned this during my life-changing hysterectomy. So then began a series of treatments, some of which were effective, and some that were not.

By doing research online, I discovered a surgeon in LA who dealt with lymphedema patients. Consequently, I had lymphatic liposuction performed and also a lymph node transfer from my right armpit to my left thigh. Both procedures were very helpful, especially removing 3.5 pounds of adipose tissue from my leg! I have followed a strict regimen of prescription compression hose, elevation, wearing a padded compression garment at night, lots of exercise, MLD massage, yoga, and a modified ketogenic diet. Keeping my BMI to 19-20 has been really beneficial.

By "modified ketogenic diet", I mean lots of protein, vegetables, and a few carbs. Although I have continued to be very active with cycling, skiing and swimming, I still lost 14-15 pounds when I went low carb. The size of my lymphedema leg went down and has been easier to manage. Then three years ago, I had my last surgery in Dallas: another lymph node transfer, this time from my abdomen to my left calf.

There are many keys to keeping lymphedema in check. Through my journey, I have discovered that it requires a LOT of work and discipline. Compression garments, elevation, wrapping, MLD, hard exercise, yoga, a healthy diet, low body weight, surgery, and most of all, a positive attitude, have allowed me to keep my stock market-looking graph at an optimal range. I am so thankful for all of the doctors, nurses, therapists, instructors and others who have helped me to maintain a great quality of life at age 67.

David D.

Obesity/Lymphedema/Weight Loss or Death

When I was asked by the author of this book to say a few things about lymphedema, two words came to mind: *bad* and *suffering*. My journey started at the age of 47 when I dislocated my knee playing football on the 4th of July. I am now 75 years old and lymphedema has changed my whole life up until now.

Five years after my injury, I had knee surgery and developed my first blood clot causing major damage in my left leg. I soon developed post-thrombotic syndrome (chronic swelling in my lower leg). The first time my leg began to swell, I did nothing. Then within several months, I suffered my second blood clot in my left thigh and I started on the blood thinner Coumadin.

When I had my first blood clot, I weighed 175 pounds and had a six-pack stomach. By the time the second clot occurred, I weighed 250 pounds prompting me to retire at 59 years old. Over the next one and a half decades, I went through repeated hospitalizations for septic blood infections, additional blood clots, pulmonary embolism and pneumonia. My weight continued to climb until I was over 400 pounds I just kept gaining and gaining.

My left leg gradually kept getting worse and soon I also had swelling in my right leg. I could not reach below my knees, so my beautiful wife had to wash my lower legs and feet and apply lotion. I had begun to see changes in my skin, particularly on my left leg with raised bumpy skin, discoloration and wounds. I saw six different doctors about the swelling and discoloration in my left leg including a pain specialist and several vein specialists and none were able to help me. I had shortness of breath and I was sleeping in a recliner chair for less than 4 hours each night. I started falling asleep at the wheel, so now my lovely wife also had to do all of the driving. I couldn't lose weight and felt bad all of the time. Eventually, I gave up on life and doctors. At this low point in my life, I was referred to Leslyn Keith who informed me I had lymphedema. I was impressed with her knowledge and her explanation of how she would treat it. At first, I was very skeptical and thought, "Here we go again." The treatment consisted of massage, wrapping both legs, and ordering special compression socks. When I had bandages on my legs, I felt like a mummy but for the first time in a very long time, my legs felt comfortable. To my surprise, my swelling started going down but still had a long way to go. This was the first time in many years of suffering that a treatment seemed to be working and my legs actually felt good. I was on my way to recovery.

In the next two years, I took two separate courses with Leslyn and learned about keto and low carbohydrate diets. Both times I lost weight, but I wasn't as successful as I needed to be. Then in October of 2019, I woke up one morning and I said to myself "What are you doing? You might be dead by Christmas 2020 and your family and friends will remember you as a person who did not try to live by losing weight!" I wanted to set an example that anyone can lose weight if they care about themselves and all those that they love.

I implemented an eating plan that I felt I could continue with for the rest of my life. I eat fewer carbohydrates and have eliminated things like sodas and juice. I only eat twice a day with smaller portions and drink more water. I don't feel hungry so I don't feel any urge to eat more food or more often. My wife and I eat out less often and we focus on eating real whole foods rather than packaged.

After nine months, my weight is 346 pounds (a loss of 68 pounds) and I am able to sleep each night between 6-8 hours. I have more energy and I don't fall asleep during the day. I am now remembering things that I learned long ago and I'm applying those skills to my everyday life more often. My blood pressure is down but most importantly, my right leg is now normal and my left leg is almost there. My skin is much better with less discoloration, smoother skin and no wounds. Even better, I can reach my feet and can take care of myself without depending on my wife. My goal now is to lose another 175 pounds in the next one and half years. I feel much more hopeful and know that I can achieve my goals and have a happy life again.

Kelly B.

While serving in the US Coast Guard in May of 2005, I had a simple medical procedure for a hiatal hernia and acid reflux called ENTERYX. ENTERYX was a liquid polymer bulking agent that was injected endoscopically at the lower esophageal sphincter to close off the hernia.

It was performed in less than 30 minutes and I was sent on my way and a month later I was deployed for my last time to Iraq.

After a few weeks, I would occasionally cough up plastic and started dealing with chest pain. Doctors checked my heart and back to work I went. A few more weeks later, I noticed I was gaining weight, especially in my trunk. I finished my deployment and came home and was transferred to Coast Guard HQ in Washington, DC and continued going to doctors for chest pain, weight gain, and just overall not feeling well.

I finally discovered in 2007 that the ENTERYX procedure had been pulled off the market due to a high risk for adverse events like my own. I received a CT Scan where I was told the polymer was *everywhere*. It was in my liver, spleen, right lung, a large chunk in the

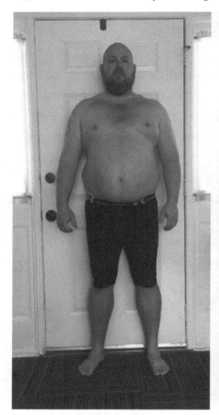
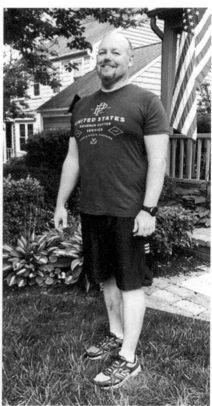

Kelly B. before keto   *Kelly B. 2 years on keto*

center of my chest, around my intestines, and in the lymph nodes at the top of my stomach. I required surgery to remove the middle lobe of my right lung. One lymph node in my chest became so engorged with polymer it exploded, spraying the polymer all over my bronchial tubes and heart. Much of the polymer can't be removed, so it still sits there today.

The surgery was not curative and it did not take long before it was apparent to me that I was not well. Over the next few years, I developed issues with my kidneys, liver, lungs, and gastrointestinal tract along with neuropathy in my arms and legs. I continued to get larger and was diagnosed as obese. In October of 2010, after developing pitting edema in my legs, arms, and the right side of my head, I was given upper and lower lymphoscintigraphies which showed "significant blockage in the area of the cisterna chyli" in my thoracic duct (correlating to polymer on CT scans). I was finally diagnosed with lymphedema all over my entire body.

The diagnosis opened the door for MLD treatments and compression garments, but nothing really led to improving my lymphedema or all of myriad other medical conditions that slowly continued to get worse. In March of 2013, I was forced to medically retire after more than 25 years of military service, in order to continue my medical struggle. My pulmonary issues progressed to the point where I was put on oxygen and I developed stage 3 congestive heart failure. It became extremely difficult to walk even a mile, let alone the athletic events I used to compete in, because of the lack of oxygen, difficulty in breathing, and neuropathy in my legs.

I had officially shifted from a participant to a spectator in my family's life. My life consisted of continuous medical visits to varying specialists, emergency rooms, and my primary care doctor. The only solution I was ever provided for improvement in my lymphedema and other medical conditions was for me to lose weight and exercise. When I showed one of the specialists that my daily diet was a 1200 calorie vegetarian diet, the recommendation was that now I just needed to work out more. It just was not possible. I continued to visit doctors and to dig through medical research on my own in a desperate effort to find answers and help for over 10 years until I finally had to acknowledge that the medical community really did not have any answers.

In January 2017, after reading through multiple medical research papers, I decided to change my diet to a ketogenic way of eating. The results for me were almost immediate. Within the first week, I lost over 9 pounds and felt like I could finally take a deep breath. I went for an evening one-mile walk and ended up walking three miles for the first time in years. In the first month, I lost over 33 pounds and knew I no longer needed supplemental oxygen. Following a strict ketogenic diet along with a strict compliance to MLD, and using my pneumatic pump, has allowed me to remove and maintain the loss of over 100 pounds of lymphatic fluid from my body. Amazingly, all my medical conditions have greatly improved, and some have disappeared. I still

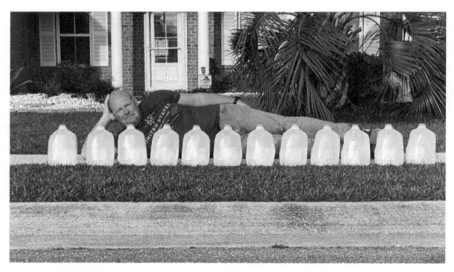

Kelly: 12 gallons of fluid lost after using a ketogenic diet.

deal with some pulmonary issues and pain due to my lymphedema but I have been able to participate in life again. I also still have "flare ups" but I can get the fluid off relatively quickly compared to the past.

I have remained strict keto for over four years. My life is not dominated by medical visits today and I don't expect it to be in the future. I also remain shocked how a modification in my diet, one that was not supported by any medical professional I was seeing at that time or even now, has had such a dramatic improvement in my health and life.

Linda P.

"Being alive is the most fun thing I have ever done."

We've all heard that diets don't work, but secretly, we know they do. It's just that we cheat on the diet, and know we are really cheating on our commitment to ourselves. Ouch! But it's true.

In 2018 I had a double mastectomy because I had breast cancer for the 2nd time, 17 years apart. The first time, I had a lumpectomy. The second time, I wanted those bitches gone!

I think they did the surgery with a bulldozer. I didn't heal well and they pulled the tubes, post surgery way too early. So I went through 6 months of drainage with tubes exiting my skin and pounds hanging from my belt. It was awful.

The best and only good thing about my adventure was that it led me to Leslyn Keith. Sweet Mercy! My Lymph System was damaged and confused. With her massage, she taught it what direction to travel and taught me how to deal with it. Because I was/am overweight, she suggested going on the Keto diet.

I have been on this diet for over a year and it is the healthiest diet I have ever been on. It starts out being very gratifying and then things slow down a bit. But by now you know how to use this way of eating and you are feeling pretty good about your results.

So you walk one more time around the block or pedal one more lap. Shazam! You are losing weight again. So you renew your commitment and now you are fitting into "those thinner clothes." Oh boy, now you can wear that darling little dress to the wedding you were just invited to! Oh my! Just look at all that food you shouldn't eat! But this is a special occasion, right? So bring on the cake, champagne, canapés, wedding candy and more champagne.

The next morning you step on the scale and… up 1~2 pounds! That's all. This is a very forgiving diet. You just get right back on your now established way of eating and here comes your gratification. You start losing again. Besides, you don't have wedding cake or canapés in your refrigerator. You only have your good stuff. And your bike wants to go for a ride.

I can tell when I've been naughty. First thing out of bed in the morning it feels like I have a baseball in each armpit. It takes extra massage and door jam exercises to make them go away. I will admit that I have yo-yo'd on more than one occasion. Certainly by now I should have reached my goal. So yes, I am weak. **But the diet doesn't hold a grudge. It is there waiting to work for you.** It is my body that punishes me with the muffin top over my jeans, my chipmunk cheeks and making me feel like I've been hit by a truck ~ and those baseballs. But when you are good, it is a wonderful diet and it makes you feel well because you are eating and shopping in a healthy way.

At this point I have only 10 pounds to lose to reach my goal. I have lost almost 50 pounds! And let's not forget that muscle weighs more than fat. So while I have been losing fat, I have been doing exercises that make me Strong, both in my core and appendages.

So yes, I should have reached my goal by now but I am what some people consider "old." And so I indulge and forgive myself. As they say, "time flies" and I am rolling downhill with no brakes. I have never been ketogenic on this diet, but I know it is working for me and giving me a healthy life. So give it a try. It may be your new way of eating without feeling deprived.

I can't give it credit for making me feel "good," because I am on a dreadful pill, post cancer for 5 years. But instead of feeling like I have been trampled by a herd of horses, it is more like a herd of ponies.

Traci J.

In June of 1981, I had a severe asthma attack while I was already a patient in the hospital for pneumonia. From that hospital visit, I was placed on a high dosage of prednisone. I remember 40 or 50 mg and taking it daily. By the end of the summer, my arms were so fat they had stretch marks. I also remember while it was still pretty warm outside, I would wear a t-shirt over a long sleeved shirt to cover up my fat arms and stretch marks. My friends would always ask me if I was hot wearing a long sleeved polyester shirt in the summertime and of course I would say NO! At this point, I hated summer.

After I graduated from high school, I went off to college and before I could finish school, I was pregnant and had my son at the age of 19 and it was a difficult pregnancy. I suffered four miscarriages between the ages of 23 and 31. By this time, not only were my arms fat, but my thighs and breasts were as well. My stomach? Not so much. At 33, I was working for an insurance company and the office attire was suits, dresses and skirts. I would wear my dresses and skirts at the knee or just a little below it. One day while in the ladies' room, a co-worker commented on how "big" my legs/calves were. I hadn't noticed and no one ever brought it to my attention. I went home and put on a pair of shorts and asked my husband what he thought and he didn't think they were too big, they looked fine to him. Even so, since that day, I don't wear shorts, skirts or dresses that would show my calves. That was 20 years ago.

Over the years I started having pains in my leg and calf area and I thought it was a blood clot but the results would always come back negative. Thank God! When I was 44, I had to have a hysterectomy and my weight had ballooned up to 307 pounds. So that same year, I decided to have gastric bypass surgery, but the lowest weight I could get to was 252 pounds The weight in my arms and calves remained. I did realize after that surgery that I was a carb junkie. Three days after the by-pass, I could have killed someone for some chips and salsa!

A year later in 2013, I started getting swelling in my right foot and legs. I went to a vein clinic and was told it wasn't a vein issue, that it looked like I have *lymphedema*, which is by the way, *incurable*. So in 2014, I began going to a lymphedema clinic for treatments. The nurse said the lymphedema was most prominent in my left leg.

After my scheduled therapies at the lymphedema clinic, I received a pump that I used for about a month and didn't use it again until 2018. After moving to Arizona in December of 2017, I began having a lot of pain and swelling in both legs. By January, my legs were so swollen they felt like they were going to pop. So that's when I began using my leg pump again for a short time. My husband also bought me a rebounder that I began using daily. I started losing weight, especially in my hips, but it seemed that my thighs were getting larger and lumpier.

In December 2018, I had my ovaries removed after a cancer scare. Then in May of 2020, I went to the Mayo Clinic for lymphedema, swelling in both legs, swelling in my right foot and shooting pain in my left thigh. I was scheduled to see a surgeon, not a lymphedema doctor. He looked me over then asked me to come back to do a scan called a lymphoscintigraphy. I scheduled the 4-hour test in June and a few hours later I had my appointment with the surgeon again. He told me at that time that the scan showed no signs of lymph blockage and that there is nothing else he can do for me. Of course I was happy that I didn't have lymph blockage, but I sat there in shock. The words fell from my mouth, but nothing from my voice. All I could say was what do you mean? Can you tell me why my legs and right foot swell all the time? He said, "I see that you wear compression stockings, maybe you need some new ones. Just order more compression and start eating right to lose weight." I'm very disappointed in how he just left me hanging with me saying, "Really I don't have lymphedema? Then what's wrong with me and my legs?" And then his response of "just exercise and eat right." He didn't even tell me that it looked like lipedema even though I read that information in his clinical notes on the patient portal. I felt like I was just dumped from a bad relationship...with no closure.

Then in September of 2020, I discovered the Keto Way of Eating for Lipedema Facebook page and my whole life has changed. On October 13, 2020, my husband also surprised me with a vibration plate! I couldn't last more than two minutes the first time on it. The Facebook group referred me to a great doctor here in Arizona [Adam Nally, DO] who has actually written a book on a keto way of eating. I began keto the day after my appointment and have lost 32 pounds! I weighed 268 pounds that first day in his office and as of today [four months later], I weigh 236 pounds.

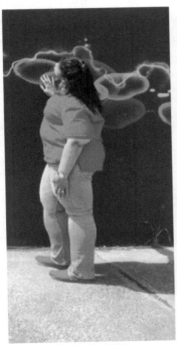
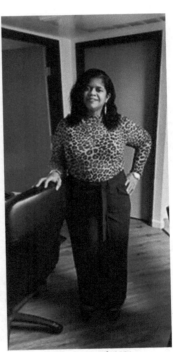

Traci - Sept 2020   *Traci - March 2021*

I just feel so much better overall. He listens, reacts and follows up. My thyroid levels, estrogen, and progesterone levels were all out of whack! But now my levels are so much better. My progesterone level was so low, it wasn't detected. I'm sleeping better, no more hot flashes! I have energy to do lymphatic yoga in the morning, jump on my rebounder for 10 minutes and get on my vibration plate for 15 minutes, all before going to work! I have better compression garments now. My old garments may have contributed to my swelling. Now I don't have swelling in my legs and feet and no longer have shooting pain in my thigh.

I have been on many diets and diet pills throughout the years. I lived off of diet pills for a long time until recently being a patient of Dr. Nally's and following keto. I wasn't losing weight, I kept taking them to keep me awake throughout the day. The diets I've tried were Atkins, the Cabbage soup diet, the Green Smoothie diet, intermittent fasting (I'm still doing this daily 16:8), and vegetarian/vegan just before keto. None of these have given me the results I have received from keto.

Traci's Results	Sept 2020		March 2021	
	just prior to keto		4 months later	
Measurement	Left leg	Right leg	Left leg	Right leg
mid-calf	23"	23.25"	20.25"	21"
lower calf	16"	14.5"	13.5"	13"

David W.

I would like to share my life-long journey with primary lymphedema and the effect changing my diet had on it. I have survived over 70 years with primary lymphedema. The name Primary Lymphedema denotes from birth. So yes, I was born with the condition of Lymphedema. The effects of lymphedema are located on my lower extremities, my legs, below the knees and my feet.

In my younger years I didn't have the benefit of health care in any form and came to realize that I was stuck with this condition for the rest of my life. Fortunately, I have an optimistic view on life and have learned to deal with it. My lymphedema wasn't too noticeable in my early years. It became more noticeable from junior high through high school. In school I always wore long pants, but it was in the gym where we all wore shorts, which is when the problems started. Whenever a person looks different, oftentimes they get picked on or teased for looking different. I put up with that during my teenage years. I'd like to think it didn't affect me, but in retrospect, it truly did. I was shy yet I had no difficulty making friends. I joined the school band and as some may know, we were all a bunch of nerds. The band was a good experience.

Wearing pants was always a problem however as clothing styles changed, I was able to adapt, starting in the 60's with Bell bottoms or in the 90's with baggies. And don't get me started on shoes. Like quadruple E's. Nothing ever fit right. While growing up I loved sports but running was my least favorite thing to do, as it was difficult. I enjoyed hiking, backpacking, swimming, which was the most fun but most of all scuba diving. Scuba diving was like visiting another planet as there was nowhere else like it. I also liked skiing, and that's where another problem occurred. I had trouble putting on ski boots due to the swelling in my feet and ankles. I solved this problem by elevating my legs all night prior to getting up and then as soon as I woke up, I quickly got dressed and put the boots on. It was still troublesome, but patience was the trick.

When I turned 21, I realized, to enjoy all these fun activities, I needed a way to pay for them. So, I got a job learning how to paint houses. This was no ordinary job either. The man who hired me was from the old country, Norway, and he started as an apprentice and worked his way up to a Master Painter. He knew everything there was to know about painting and wallpaper. That job is what led me to become a painting contractor.

Painting houses is one of the toughest jobs, but the rewards are great. I painted houses for 40 years and during that time there were personal struggles with my lymphedema. There are unseen dangers in my profession. On one job, I hit a sharp metal edge of a bed frame which made a gash in my leg, blood flowed quickly followed by lymph fluid. I found that injuries such as these take months to heal because of the constant flow of lymph fluid. Over the years I had several injuries similar to this one and became very adept at treating them.

The painting business also involves a lot of ladder work. Climbing ladders all day is that much harder when your legs have the added weight of lymph fluid that just stays in your legs, creates swelling, and doesn't circulate. The older I got the less I seemed to accomplish. I was doing all this work solo. It's a good thing that I loved painting so much, I probably would have found something else.

When I was finally able to afford insurance and discovered there were clinics that could actually treat people with my lymphatic condition I was elated. I found a clinic in San Luis Obispo near where I live and made an appointment. It's where I met Leslyn Keith. At my first visit, Leslyn suggested that I try to follow a ketogenic way of eating prior to any treatment for my lymphedema, as I was extremely overweight. She explained to me about Dr. Eric Westman and page 4. I took her advice and after leaving her office, went home and listened to everything I could about Dr. Eric Westman. I joined the LCHF Facebook group and got a copy of page 4.

After about 5 or 6 months I returned to Leslyn's office and she discovered that I had lost 50 pounds and my legs were already smaller. So that is when treatment started for my lymphedema. I was 65 years old. The treatment took 6 weeks and the swelling in my legs had been reduced by almost 50 percent which I was pleasantly surprised. I continued with my keto lifestyle and after 14 months I lost a total of 80 pounds. I maintained the weight loss for 1-2 years and during that time I really enjoyed the new me, lighter and able to do things with greater ease. After all, I was a painting contractor for 40 years and going up and down ladders can be grueling at times. Now that I had more energy, work came easier.

The older I got the more I started thinking about retiring and all of a sudden, the answer became clear. I fell off my scaffolding and ended up in the hospital, followed five days later by being transferred to transitional care where I stayed for 37 days. I had broken my pelvis and other injuries to my back. During my stay at this facility, I found that their food was prepared fresh every day, if you had a diet preference, they would prepare it as ordered. I was able to maintain my way of eating, which was a blessing.

There was one issue that occurred each night at 9 pm. The kitchen staff would roll a dessert cart past every room with offerings of fresh baked cakes and ice cream, cookies, brownies. It was a temptation that I managed to stand up to for at least three weeks of my stay. However, a person can only take so much, and I finally broke down and started sampling the goods. Just like that I was a goner. When I was finally released from the facility, I was off my eating regimen and eating whatever. I must say that being on LCHF [low carb high fat] way of eating is ingrained into my mind and I'm always conscious of what I should be eating, just not following the program I set for myself.

One benefit from San Luis Transitional Care, I rolled in there on a stretcher and walked out with a walker. The therapists were and are wonderful and motivating. I occasionally stop back by there to visit and chat. They appreciate the visit. I left the transitional care facility in October of 2017 and went home. I experienced in-home physical therapy and after about three months and a difficult time of weaning myself off pain meds, I was able to function semi-normally. In the back of my mind, I really wanted to get back to work painting, probably in a limited fashion, yet at least I'd be doing something.

During this time, I was trying to eat low carb and sweets. That idea wasn't working too well. It took me three years to finally get back to feeling normal. After three years I had gained about 60 pounds back. I came to a decision at the end of July 2020 to get serious about LCHF. Once again, I started my way of eating and never looked back. Today, I've lost 35 pounds and am on the road to success, which is a good feeling. Like all things difficult, with perseverance anything can be accomplished. Just don't give up and have a positive attitude!

References

1. Granger, D. N., Skeff, K. M., Chaite, W. & Rockson, S. G. Lymphatic biology and disease: Is it being taught? Who Is listening? *Lymphat. Res. Biol.* **2**, 86–95 (2004).

2. Rockson, S. G. Lymphatic Medicine: Paradoxically and unnecessarily ignored. *Lymphat. Res. Biol.* **15**, 315–316 (2017).

3. Choi, I., Lee, S. & Hong, Y.-K. The new era of the lymphatic system: No longer secondary to the blood vascular system. *Cold Spring Harb. Perspect. Med.* **2**, a006445 (2012).

4. Natale, G., Bocci, G. & Ribatti, D. Scholars and scientists in the history of the lymphatic system. *J. Anat.* **231**, 417–429 (2017).

5. Loukas, M. *et al.* The lymphatic system: A historical perspective. *Clin. Anat.* **24**, 807–816 (2011).

6. Starling, E. H. On the absorption of fluids from the connective tissue spaces. *J. Physiol.* **19**, 312–326 (1896).

7. Levick, J. R. & Michel, C. C. Microvascular fluid exchange and the revised Starling principle. *Cardiovasc. Res.* **87**, 198–210 (2010).

8. Koltowska, K., Betterman, K. L., Harvey, N. L. & Hogan, B. M. Getting out and about: The emergence and morphogenesis of the vertebrate lymphatic vasculature. *Development* **140**, 1857–1870 (2013).

9. Yaniv, K. *et al.* Live imaging of lymphatic development in the zebrafish. *Nat. Med.* **12**, 711–716 (2006).

10. Casley-Smith, J. *Modern Treatment for Lymphoedema.* (The Lymphoedema Association of Australia, Inc, 1997).

11. von der Weid, P.-Y. & Zawieja, D. C. Lymphatic smooth muscle: The motor unit of lymph drainage. *Int. J. Biochem. Cell Biol.* **36**, 1147–1153 (2004).

12. Aukland, K. & Reed, R. K. Interstitial-lymphatic mechanisms in the control of extracellular fluid volume. *Physiol. Rev.* **73**, 1–78 (1993).

13. Moriondo, A., Mukenge, S. & Negrini, D. Transmural pressure in rat initial subpleural lymphatics during spontaneous or mechanical ventilation. *Am. J. Physiol.-Heart Circ. Physiol.* **289**, H263–H269 (2005).

14. Hedrick, M. S., Hillman, S. S., Drewes, R. C. & Withers, P. C. Lymphatic regulation in nonmammalian vertebrates. *J. Appl. Physiol.* **115**, 297–308 (2013).

15. Butler, M. G., Isogai, S. & Weinstein, B. M. Lymphatic development. *Birth Defects Res. Part C Embryo Today Rev.* **87**, 222–231 (2009).

16. Oliver, G., Kipnis, J., Randolph, G. & Harvey, N. The lymphatic vasculature in the 21st century: Novel functional roles in homeostasis and disease. *Cell* **182**, 270–296 (2020).

17. Pond, M. & Mattacks, A. Interactions between adipose tissue around lymph nodes and lymphoid cells in vitro. *J. Lipid Res.* **36**, 2219–31 (1995).

18. Hausman, D. B., DiGirolamo, M., Bartness, T. J., Hausman, G. J. & Martin, R. J. The biology of white adipocyte proliferation. *Obes. Rev.* **2**, 239–254 (2001).

19. Pond C.M. (2017) The Evolution of Mammalian Adipose Tissues. In: Symonds M. (eds) *Adipose Tissue Biology.* Springer, Cham. https://doi.org/10.1007/978-3-319-52031-5_1.

20. Petrova, T. V. & Koh, G. Y. Organ-specific lymphatic vasculature: From development to pathophysiology. *J. Exp. Med.* **215**, 35–49 (2018).

21. Jakus, Z. *et al.* Lymphatic function is required prenatally for lung inflation at birth. *J. Exp. Med.* **211**, 815–826 (2014).

22. Angeli, V. & Harvey, N. L. Lymphatic vessels at the heart of the matter. *Cell Metab.* **22**, 56–58 (2015).

23. Sabin, F. R. On the origin of the lymphatic system from the veins and the development of the lymph hearts and thoracic duct in the pig. *Am. J. Anat.* **1**, 367–389 (1902).

24. Butler, E. G. Charles Freeman Williams McClure. *Anat. Rec.* **126**, 129–142 (1956).

25. Cueni, L. N. & Detmar, M. The lymphatic system in health and disease. *Lymphat. Res. Biol.* **6**, 109–122 (2008).

26. Oliver, G. & Detmar, M. The rediscovery of the lymphatic system: Old and new insights into the development and biological function of the lymphatic vasculature. *Genes Dev.* **16**, 773–783 (2002).

27. Nakamura, K. & Rockson, S. G. Biomarkers of lymphatic function and disease: State of the art and future directions. *Mol. Diagn. Ther.* **11**, 227–238 (2007).

28. García-Caballero, M. *et al.* Role and therapeutic potential of dietary ketone bodies in lymph vessel growth. *Nat. Metab.* **1**, 666–675 (2019).

29. Wong, B. W. *et al.* The role of fatty acid β-oxidation in lymphangiogenesis. *Nature* **542**, 49–54 (2017).

30. Jensen, G. L. *et al.* Dietary modification of chyle composition in chylothorax. *Gastroenterology* **97**, 761–765 (1989).

31. Goss, J. A., Maclellan, R. A., Beijnen, U. E. A. & Greene, A. K. Resolution of primary lymphedema: A case report. *Plast. Reconstr. Surg. Glob. Open* **5**, (2017).

32. Mejia, E. J. *et al.* Use of contrast-enhanced ultrasound to determine thoracic duct patency. *J. Vasc. Interv. Radiol.* **31**, 1670–1674 (2020).

33. Munn, L. & Padera, T., Imaging the lymphatic system. *Microvasc. Res.* **96**, 55–63 (2014).

34. Guermazi, A., Brice, P., Hennequin, C. & Sarfati, E. Lymphography: An old technique retains its usefulness. *RadioGraphics* **23**, 1541–1558 (2003).

35. Biko, D. M. *et al.* Intrahepatic dynamic contrast MR lymphangiography: Initial experience with a new technique for the assessment of liver lymphatics. *Eur. Radiol.* **29**, 5190–5196 (2019).

36. Suami, H. *et al.* A new indocyanine green fluorescence lymphography protocol for identification of the lymphatic drainage pathway for patients with breast cancer-related lymphoedema. *BMC Cancer* **19**, 985 (2019).

37. Louveau, A. *et al.* Structural and functional features of central nervous system lymphatics. *Nature* **523**, 337–341 (2015).

38. Yang, A. Playing it by ear: Investigating the role of the inner ear in lymphatic development. (ResearchSpace@Auckland, 2020).

39. Rudzki, Z. *et al.* Fatal systemic angiomatosis with widespread sclerotic skeletal changes, diagnosed with the aid of a bone marrow biopsy: The lymphatics enter the bone marrow. *Pol. J. Pathol.* **69**, 314–318 (2018).

40. Ozeki, M. *et al.* Clinical features and prognosis of generalized lymphatic anomaly, Kaposiform lymphangiomatosis, and Gorham–Stout disease. *Pediatr. Blood Cancer* **63**, 832–838 (2016).

41. Chang, L.-R., O'Connell, K. & Martin, A. Anatomy, Cartilage. in *StatPearls* (StatPearls Publishing, 2020).

42. Reitsma, S., Slaaf, D. W., Vink, H., van Zandvoort, M. A. M. J. & oude Egbrink, M. G. A. The endothelial glycocalyx: Composition, functions, and visualization. *Pflugers Arch.* **454**, 345–359 (2007).

43. Nieuwdorp, M. *et al.* Loss of endothelial glycocalyx during acute hyperglycemia coincides with endothelial dysfunction and coagulation activation in vivo. *Diabetes* **55**, 480–486 (2006).

44. Moore, J. E. & Bertram, C. D. Lymphatic system flows. *Annu. Rev. Fluid Mech.* **50**, 459–482 (2018).

45. Scallan, J. P., Hill, M. A. & Davis, M. J. Lymphatic vascular integrity is disrupted in type 2 diabetes due to impaired nitric oxide signalling. *Cardiovasc. Res.* **107**, 89–97 (2015).

46. Margaris, K. N. & Black, R. A. Modelling the lymphatic system: Challenges and opportunities. *J. R. Soc. Interface* **9**, 601–612 (2012).

47. Zolla, V. *et al.* Aging-related anatomical and biochemical changes in lymphatic collectors impair lymph transport, fluid homeostasis, and pathogen clearance. *Aging Cell* **14**, 582–594 (2015).

48. Davis, M. J. *et al.* Intrinsic increase in lymphangion muscle contractility in response to elevated afterload. *Am. J. Physiol.-Heart Circ. Physiol.* **303**, H795–H808 (2012).

49. Harvey, N. L. The link between lymphatic function and adipose biology. *Ann. N. Y. Acad. Sci.* **1131**, 82–88 (2008).

50. Johnson, O. W. *et al.* The thoracic duct: Clinical importance, anatomic variation, imaging, and embolization. *Eur. Radiol.* **26**, 2482–2493 (2016).

51. Hsu, M. C. & Itkin, M. Lymphatic anatomy. *Tech. Vasc. Interv. Radiol.* **19**, 247–254 (2016).

52. Mortimer, P. S. & Levick, J. R. Chronic peripheral oedema: The critical role of the lymphatic system. *Clin. Med.* **4**, 448–453 (2004).

53. Hareyama, H. *et al.* Prevalence, classification, and risk factors for postoperative lower extremity lymphedema in women with gynecologic malignancies: A retrospective study. *Int. J. Gynecol. Cancer* **25**, 751–757 (2015).

54. Collin, M. & Bigley, V. Human dendritic cell subsets: An update. *Immunology* **154**, 3–20 (2018).

55. Arasa, J. *et al.* Upregulation of VCAM-1 in lymphatic collectors supports dendritic cell entry and rapid migration to lymph nodes in inflammation. *J. Exp. Med.* **218**, (2021).

56. Sriram, K., Meguid, R. A. & Meguid, M. M. Nutritional support in adults with chyle leaks. *Nutrition* **32**, 281–286 (2016).

57. Heffner, JE. Etiology, clinical presentation, and diagnosis of chylothorax – UpToDate. https://www-uptodate-com.ezproxy.lib.utah.edu/contents/etiology-clinical-presentation-and-diagnosis-of-chylothorax.

58. McCray, S. & Parrish, C. R. Nutritional management of chyle leaks: An update. *Pract. Gastroenterol.* 13 (2011).

59. Huang, L.-H., Elvington, A. & Randolph, G. J. The role of the lymphatic system in cholesterol transport. *Front. Pharmacol.* **6**, (2015).

60. Gardenier, J. C. *et al.* Topical tacrolimus for the treatment of secondary lymphedema. *Nat. Commun.* **8**, 14345 (2017).

61. Ma, W. *et al.* Platelet factor 4 is a biomarker for lymphatic-promoted disorders. *JCI Insight* (2020) doi:10.1172/jci.insight.135109.

62. Brorson, H. Liposuction in lymphedema treatment. *J. Reconstr. Microsurg.* **32**, 56–65 (2016).

63. Deng, J. *et al.* Factors associated with reported infection and lymphedema symptoms among individuals with extremity lymphedema. *Rehabil. Nurs.* **40**, 310–319 (2015).

64. Carlson, J. A. Lymphedema and subclinical lymphostasis (microlymphedema) facilitate cutaneous infection, inflammatory dermatoses, and neoplasia: A locus minoris resistentiae. *Clin. Dermatol.* **32**, 599–615 (2014).

65. Ibrahim, M., Zambruni, M., Melby, C. & Melby, P. Impact of childhood malnutrition on host defense and infection. *Clin. Microbiol. Rev.* **30**, 919–971 (2017).

66. Fu, M. R. *et al.* Psychosocial impact of lymphedema: A systematic review of literature from 2004 to 2011. *Psychooncology.* **22**, 1466–1484 (2013).

67. Stolldorf, D. P., Dietrich, M. S. & Ridner, S. H. A comparison of the quality of life in patients with primary and secondary lower limb lymphedema: A mixed-methods study. *West. J. Nurs. Res.* **38**, 1313–1334 (2016).

68. Lee, T. S., Morris, C. M., Czerniec, S. A. & Mangion, A. J. Does lymphedema severity affect quality of life? Simple question. Challenging answers. *Lymphat. Res. Biol.* **16**, 85–91 (2017).

69. Klose, G. Complete Decongestive Therapy Reimagined. Power Lymphatics 2021 Virtual Conference (2021).

70. Armer, J. M. *et al.* Lymphedema within the healthcare system. in *Lymphedema: A Concise Compendium of Theory and Practice* (eds. Lee, B.-B., Rockson, S. G. & Bergan, J.) 503–523 (Springer International Publishing, 2018). doi:10.1007/978-3-319-52423-8_40.

71. Ozmen, T., Lazaro, M., Zhou, Y., Vinyard, A. & Avisar, E. Evaluation of Simplified Lymphatic Microsurgical Preventing Healing Approach (S-LYMPHA) for the prevention of breast cancer–related clinical lymphedema after axillary lymph node dissection. *Ann. Surg.* **270**, 1156–1160 (2019).

72. Wold, L., Hines, E. & Allen. Lipedema of the legs: A syndrome characterized by fat legs and edema. *Ann. Intern. Med.* **34**, 1243 (1951).

73. Bertsch, T. & Erbacher, G. Lipödem – mythen und fakten teil 1. (2018) doi:10.12687/PHLEB2411-2-2018.

74. Lohrmann, C., Foeldi, E. & Langer, M. MR imaging of the lymphatic system in patients with lipedema and lipo-lymphedema. *Microvasc. Res.* **77**, 335–339 (2009).

75. Forner-Cordero, I., Szolnoky, G., Forner-Cordero, A. & Kemény, L. Lipedema: An overview of its clinical manifestations, diagnosis and treatment of the disproportional fatty deposition syndrome – Systematic review. *Clin. Obes.* **2**, 86–95 (2012).

76. Gould, D. J. *et al.* Uncovering lymphatic transport abnormalities in patients with primary lipedema. *J. Reconstr. Microsurg.* **36**, 136–141 (2020).

77. Fife, C. E., Maus, E. A. & Carter, M. J. Lipedema: A frequently misdiagnosed and misunderstood fatty deposition syndrome. *Adv. Skin Wound Care* **23**, 81–92 (2010).

78. Herbst, K. L., Mirkovskaya, L., Bharhagava, A., Chava, Y. & Te, C. H. T. Lipedema fat and signs and symptoms of illness, increase with advancing stage. *Arch. Med.* **7**, 8 (2015).

79. Child, A. H. *et al.* Lipedema: An inherited condition. *Am. J. Med. Genet. A.* **152A**, 970–976 (2010).

80. Rapprich, S., Dingler, A. & Podda, M. Liposuction is an effective treatment for lipedema–results of a study with 25 patients. *JDDG J. Dtsch. Dermatol. Ges.* **9**, 33–40 (2011).

81. Dadras, M., Mallinger, P. J., Corterier, C. C., Theodosiadi, S. & Ghods, M. Liposuction in the treatment of lipedema: A longitudinal study. *Arch. Plast. Surg.* **44**, 324–331 (2017).

82. Georgiou, I., Kruppa, P., Schmidt, J. & Ghods, M. Liposuction for lipedema: Functional therapy or aesthetic procedure? *Aesthetic Plast. Surg.* **45**, 212–213 (2021).

83. Klein, S. *et al.* Absence of an effect of liposuction on insulin action and risk factors for coronary heart disease. *N. Engl. J. Med.* **350**, 2549–2557 (2004).

84.   Hernandez, T. L. *et al.* Fat redistribution following suction lipectomy: Defense of body fat and patterns of restoration. *Obesity* **19**, 1388–1395 (2011).

85.   Executive Committee of the International Society of Lymphology. The diagnosis and treatment of peripheral lymphedema: 2020 Consensus Document of the International Society of Lymphology. *Lymphology* **53**, 3–19 (2020).

86.   Santler, B. & Goerge, T. Chronic venous insufficiency – a review of pathophysiology, diagnosis, and treatment. *JDDG J. Dtsch. Dermatol. Ges.* **15**, 538–556 (2017).

87.   Rüttermann, M., Maier-Hasselmann, A., Nink-Grebe, B. & Burckhardt, M. Local treatment of chronic wounds. *Dtsch. Ärztebl. Int.* **110**, 25–31 (2013).

88.   Coulthard, M. Oedema in kwashiorkor is caused by hypoalbuminaemia. *Paediatr. Int. Child Health* **35**, 83–89 (2015).

89.   Braamskamp, M. J. A. M., Dolman, K. M. & Tabbers, M. M. Clinical practice: Protein-losing enteropathy in children. *Eur. J. Pediatr.* **169**, 1179–1185 (2010).

90.   Honore, P. M. *et al.* Statins and the kidney: Friend or foe? *Blood Purif.* **43**, 91–96 (2017).

91.   Mudaliar, S. *et al.* Efficacy and safety of the farnesoid X receptor agonist obeticholic acid in patients with type 2 diabetes and nonalcoholic fatty liver disease. *Gastroenterology* **145**, 574-582.e1 (2013).

92.   Langsjoen, P. H. & Langsjoen, A. M. Supplemental ubiquinol in patients with advanced congestive heart failure. *BioFactors* **32**, 119–128 (2008).

93.   Zawieja, S. D. *et al.* Impairments in the intrinsic contractility of mesenteric collecting lymphatics in a rat model of metabolic syndrome. *Am. J. Physiol. – Heart Circ. Physiol.* **302**, H643–H653 (2012).

94.   Chakraborty, S., Zawieja, S., Wang, W., Zawieja, D. C. & Muthuchamy, M. Lymphatic system: A vital link between metabolic syndrome and inflammation: Roles of lymphatics in metabolic syndrome. *Ann. N. Y. Acad. Sci.* **1207**, E94–E102 (2010).

95.   Schmitz, K. H. *et al.* Effect of home-based exercise and weight loss programs on breast cancer–related lymphedema outcomes among overweight breast cancer survivors: The WISER Survivor Randomized Clinical Trial. *JAMA Oncol.* **5**, 1605–1613 (2019).

96.   Yang, Q. & Guan, K.-L. Expanding mTOR signaling. *Cell Res.* **17**, 666–681 (2007).

97.   Wiegand, S., Wichmann, G. & Dietz, A. Treatment of lymphatic malformations with the mTOR inhibitor sirolimus: A systematic review. *Lymphat. Res. Biol.* **16**, 330–339 (2018).

98.   McDaniel, S. S., Rensing, N. R., Thio, L. L., Yamada, K. A. & Wong, M. The ketogenic diet inhibits the mammalian target of rapamycin (mTOR) pathway. *Epilepsia* **52**, e7–e11 (2011).

99.   Miura, S. *et al.* Increased lymphocyte transport by lipid absorption in rat mesenteric lymphatics. *Am. J. Physiol.-Gastrointest. Liver Physiol.* **253**, G596–G600 (1987).

100. Mattacks, C. A. & Pond, C. M. Interactions of noradrenalin and tumour necrosis factor α, interleukin 4 and interleukin 6 in the control of lipolysis from adipocytes around lymph nodes. *Cytokine* **11**, 334–346 (1999).

101. Mattacks, C. A., Sadler, D. & Pond, C. M. Site-specific differences in fatty acid composition of dendritic cells and associated adipose tissue in popliteal depot, mesentery, and omentum and their modulation by chronic inflammation and dietary lipids. *Lymphat. Res. Biol.* **2**, 107–129 (2004).

102. Hausman, D. B., Lu, J., Ryan, D. H., Flatt, W. P. & Harris, R. B. S. Compensatory growth of adipose tissue after partial lipectomy: Involvement of serum factors. *Exp. Biol. Med.* **229**, 512–520 (2004).

103. Sadler, D., Mattacks, C. A. & Pond, C. M. Changes in adipocytes and dendritic cells in lymph node containing adipose depots during and after many weeks of mild inflammation. *J. Anat.* **207**, 769–781 (2005).

104. Thomis, Sarah. *Ketogenic Diet: A Novel Metabolic Strategy to Treat Lymphedema Patients?* https://clinicaltrials.gov/ct2/show/NCT03991897 (2019).

105. Rockson, S. Of Mice and Man: What Modern Research Teaches Us about Lymphatic Disease. (2020).

106. Miller, A. J. The grossly invisible and generally ignored lymphatics of the mammalian heart. *Med. Hypotheses* **76**, 604–606 (2011).

107. Mouta, C. & Heroult, M. Inflammatory triggers of lymphangiogenesis. *Lymphat. Res. Biol.* **1**, 201–218 (2003).

108. Schwager, S. & Detmar, M. Inflammation and lymphatic function. *Front. Immunol.* **10**, (2019).

109. Kim, H., Kataru, R. P. & Koh, G. Y. Inflammation-associated lymphangiogenesis: A double-edged sword? https://www.jci.org/articles/view/71607/pdf (2014) doi:10.1172/JCI71607.

110. Kajiya, K. & Detmar, M. An important role of lymphatic vessels in the control of UVB-induced edema formation and inflammation. *J. Invest. Dermatol.* **126**, 920–922 (2006).

111. Liu, X. *et al.* Lymphoangiocrine signals promote cardiac growth and repair. *Nature* **588**, 705–711 (2020).

112. Neely, J. R. & Morgan, H. E. Relationship between carbohydrate and lipid metabolism and the energy balance of heart muscle. *Annu. Rev. Physiol.* **36**, 413–459 (1974).

113. McCommis, K. S. *et al.* Nutritional modulation of heart failure in mitochondrial pyruvate carrier–deficient mice. *Nat. Metab.* (2020) doi:10.1038/s42255-020-00296-1.

114. Volek, J. S. & Feinman, R. D. Carbohydrate restriction improves the features of Metabolic Syndrome. Metabolic Syndrome may be defined by the response to carbohydrate restriction. *Nutr. Metab.* **2**, 31 (2005).

115. Caillon, A. & Schiffrin, E. L. Role of inflammation and immunity in hypertension: Recent epidemiological, laboratory, and clinical evidence. *Curr. Hypertens. Rep.* **18**, 21 (2016).

116. Dzielak, D. J. Immune mechanisms in experimental and essential hypertension. *Am. J. Physiol.-Regul. Integr. Comp. Physiol.* **260**, R459–R467 (1991).

117. Chachaj, A. *et al.* Role of the lymphatic system in the pathogenesis of hypertension in humans. *Lymphat. Res. Biol.* **16**, 140–146 (2018).

118. Titze, J. & Machnik, A. Sodium sensing in the interstitium and relationship to hypertension. *Curr. Opin. Nephrol. Hypertens.* **19**, 385–392 (2010).

119. Bueno, N. B., de Melo, I. S. V., de Oliveira, S. L. & da Rocha Ataide, T. Very-low-carbohydrate ketogenic diet vs low-fat diet for long-term weight loss: A meta-analysis of randomised controlled trials. *Br. J. Nutr.* **110**, 1178–1187 (2013).

120. Tóth, C. & Clemens, Z. Successful treatment of a patient with obesity, type 2 diabetes and hypertension with the paleolithic ketogenic diet. *Int. J. Case Rep. Images* **6**, 161 (2015).

121. Golosova, D., Levchenko, V., Spires, D., Staruschenko, A. & Palygin, O. The protective effects of ketodiet in salt-sensitive hypertension. *FASEB J.* **34**, 1–1 (2020).

122. Canto, J. G. Symptom presentation of women with acute coronary syndromes: Myth vs reality. *Arch. Intern. Med.* **167**, 2405 (2007).

123. Nakamura, K. & Rockson, S. G. The role of the lymphatic circulation in the natural history and expression of cardiovascular disease. *Int. J. Cardiol.* **129**, 309–317 (2008).

124. Maroko, P. R. *et al.* Favorable effects of hyaluronidase on electrocardiographic evidence of necrosis in patients with acute myocardial infarction. *N. Engl. J. Med.* **296**, 898–903 (1977).

125. Yotsumoto, G., Moriyama, Y., Yamaoka, A. & Taira, A. Experimental study of cardiac lymph dynamics and edema formation in ischemia/reperfusion injury— with reference to the effect of hyaluronidase. *Angiology* **49**, 299–305 (1998).

126. Brakenhielm, E. & Alitalo, K. Cardiac lymphatics in health and disease. *Nat. Rev. Cardiol.* **16**, 56–68 (2019).

127. Klotz, L. *et al.* Cardiac lymphatics are heterogeneous in origin and respond to injury. *Nature* **522**, 62–67 (2015).

128. Davis, W. *Wheat Belly: Lose the Wheat, Lose the Weight, and Find Your Path Back to Health.* (Rodale, 2011).

129. Mente, A. *et al.* Associations of urinary sodium excretion with cardiovascular events in individuals with and without hypertension: A pooled analysis of data from four studies. *The Lancet* **388**, 465–475 (2016).

130. Houck, P. Alternative view of congestive heart failure exacerbations: Role of lymphatic function and inflammation. *Med. Hypothesis* **1**, 6 (2013).

131. Houck, P., Dandapantula, H., Hardegree, E. & Massey, J. Why we fail at heart failure: Lymphatic insufficiency is disregarded. *Cureus* **12**, (2020).

132. Mortimer, P. Managing lymphedema. Clin. Dermatol. 13, 499–505 (1995).

133. Fejfarová, V. *et al.* The relationship between chronic venous insufficiency and diabetes mellitus. *Int. Angiol. J. Int. Union Angiol.* **36**, 90–91 (2017).

134. Feinman, R. D. *et al.* Dietary carbohydrate restriction as the first approach in diabetes management: Critical review and evidence base. *Nutr. Burbank Los Angel. Cty. Calif* **31**, 1–13 (2015).

135. Milasan, A., Ledoux, J. & Martel, C. Lymphatic network in atherosclerosis: The underestimated path. *Future Sci. OA* **1**, (2015).

136. Martel, C. *et al.* Lymphatic vasculature mediates macrophage reverse cholesterol transport in mice. *J. Clin. Invest.* **123**, 1571–1579 (2013).

137. Jiang, X., Tian, W., Nicolls, M. R. & Rockson, S. G. The lymphatic system in obesity, insulin resistance, and cardiovascular diseases. *Front. Physiol.* **10**, (2019).

138. Lemole, G. M. The role of lymphstasis in atherogenesis. *Ann. Thorac. Surg.* **31**, 290–293 (1981).

139. Kutkut, I., Meens, M. J., McKee, T. A., Bochaton-Piallat, M.-L. & Kwak, B. R. Lymphatic vessels: An emerging actor in atherosclerotic plaque development. *Eur. J. Clin. Invest.* **45**, 100–108 (2015).

140. Subbotin, V. M. Excessive intimal hyperplasia in human coronary arteries before intimal lipid depositions is the initiation of coronary atherosclerosis and constitutes a therapeutic target. *Drug Discov. Today* **21**, 1578–1595 (2016).

141. Sano, M. *et al.* Topologic distributions of vasa vasorum and lymphatic vasa vasorum in the aortic adventitia – Implications for the prevalence of aortic diseases. *Atherosclerosis* **247**, 127–134 (2016).

142. Johnson, L. A. & Jackson, D. G. Inflammation-induced secretion of CCL21 in lymphatic endothelium is a key regulator of integrin-mediated dendritic cell transmigration. *Int. Immunol.* **22**, 839–849 (2010).

143. Tal, O. *et al.* DC mobilization from the skin requires docking to immobilized CCL21 on lymphatic endothelium and intralymphatic crawling. *J. Exp. Med.* **208**, 2141–2153 (2011).

144. Lim, H. Y. *et al.* Lymphatic vessels are essential for the removal of cholesterol from peripheral tissues by sr-bi-mediated transport of hdl. *Cell Metab.* **17**, 671–684 (2013).

145. DeFronzo, R. A. & Tripathy, D. Skeletal muscle insulin resistance is the primary defect in type 2 diabetes. *Diabetes Care* **32**, S157–S163 (2009).

146. Li, S., Brown, M. S. & Goldstein, J. L. Bifurcation of insulin signaling pathway in rat liver: mTORC1 required for stimulation of lipogenesis, but not inhibition of gluconeogenesis. *Proc. Natl. Acad. Sci.* **107**, 3441–3446 (2010).

147. Saklayen, M. G. The global epidemic of the metabolic syndrome. *Curr. Hypertens. Rep.* **20**, (2018).

148. Sohouli, M. H. *et al.* The effect of paleolithic diet on glucose metabolism and lipid profile among patients with metabolic disorders: A systematic review and meta-analysis of randomized controlled trials. *Crit. Rev. Food Sci. Nutr.* **0**, 1–12 (2021).

149. Cifarelli, V. & Eichmann, A. The intestinal lymphatic system: Functions and metabolic implications. *Cell. Mol. Gastroenterol. Hepatol.* **7**, 503–513 (2019).

150. Norden, P. R. & Kume, T. The role of lymphatic vascular function in metabolic disorders. *Front. Physiol.* **11**, (2020).

151. Westman, E. C., Tondt, J., Maguire, E. & Jr, W. S. Y. Implementing a low-carbohydrate, ketogenic diet to manage type 2 diabetes mellitus. *Expert Rev. Endocrinol. Metab.* **13**, 263–272 (2018).

152. Athinarayanan, S. J. *et al.* 759-p: analysis of a two-year continuous care intervention including nutritional ketosis—exploring baseline predictors of diabetes reversal and remission. *Diabetes* **68**, (2019).

153. Kalambokis, G. N., Tsatsoulis, A. A. & Tsianos, E. V. The edematogenic properties of insulin. *Am. J. Kidney Dis.* **44**, 575–590 (2004).

154. Lee, Y., Chakraborty, S., Meininger, C. J. & Muthuchamy, M. Insulin resistance disrupts cell integrity, mitochondrial function, and inflammatory signaling in lymphatic endothelium. *Microcirculation* **25**, e12492 (2018).

155. Seyfried, T. Role of lymphatics in cancer metastasis. (2020).

156. Skobe, M. *et al.* Induction of tumor lymphangiogenesis by VEGF-C promotes breast cancer metastasis. Nat Med 7: 192-198. *Nat. Med.* **7**, 192–8 (2001).

157. Veronesi, U. *et al.* Sentinel lymph node biopsy in breast cancer: Ten-year results of a randomized controlled study. *Ann. Surg.* **251**, 595–600 (2010).

158. Wong, S. L. *et al.* Sentinel Lymph Node Biopsy for Melanoma: American Society of Clinical Oncology and Society of Surgical Oncology Joint Clinical Practice Guideline. *Ann. Surg. Oncol.* **19**, 3313–3324 (2012).

159. Pasquali, S. *et al.* Lymphatic biomarkers in primary melanomas as predictors of regional lymph node metastasis and patient outcomes. *Pigment Cell Melanoma Res.* **26**, 326–337 (2013).

160. Nagahashi, M., Ramachandran, S., Rashid, O. M. & Takabe, K. Lymphangiogenesis: A new player in cancer progression. *World J. Gastroenterol. WJG* **16**, 4003–4012 (2010).

161. Fankhauser, M. *et al.* Tumor lymphangiogenesis promotes T cell infiltration and potentiates immunotherapy in melanoma. *Sci. Transl. Med.* **9**, (2017).

162. Song, J. *et al.* CCBE1 promotes tumor lymphangiogenesis and is negatively regulated by TGFβ signaling in colorectal cancer. *Theranostics* **10**, 2327–2341 (2020).

163. Naxerova, K. *et al.* Origins of lymphatic and distant metastases in human colorectal cancer. *Science* **357**, 55–60 (2017).

164. Liao, S. & Padera, T. P. Lymphatic function and immune regulation in health and disease. *Lymphat. Res. Biol.* **11**, 136–143 (2013).

165. Schwartz, L., Seyfried, T., Alfarouk, K. O., Da Veiga Moreira, J. & Fais, S. Out of Warburg effect: An effective cancer treatment targeting the tumor specific metabolism and dysregulated pH. *Semin. Cancer Biol.* **43**, 134–138 (2017).

166. Weber, D. D., Aminazdeh-Gohari, S. & Kofler, B. Ketogenic diet in cancer therapy. *Aging* **10**, 164–165 (2018).

167. Szoták-Ajtay, K. *et al.* Reduced prenatal pulmonary lymphatic function is observed in clp1 k/k embryos with impaired motor functions including fetal breathing movements in preparation of the developing lung for inflation at birth. *Front. Bioeng. Biotechnol.* **8**, 136 (2020).

168. Reed, H. O. *et al.* Lymphatic impairment leads to pulmonary tertiary lymphoid organ formation and alveolar damage. *J. Clin. Invest.* **129**, 2514–2526 (2019).

169. Jung, J. I. *et al.* Mediastinal lymphadenopathy in pulmonary fibrosis: Correlation with disease severity. *J. Comput. Assist. Tomogr.* **24**, 706–710 (2000).

170. Sin, S. *et al.* Impact of mediastinal lymph node enlargement on the prognosis of idiopathic pulmonary fibrosis. *PloS One* **13**, e0201154 (2018).

171. Behr, M. A. & Waters, W. R. Is tuberculosis a lymphatic disease with a pulmonary portal? *Lancet Infect. Dis.* **14**, 250–255 (2014).

172. Uhley, H. N., Leeds, S. E., Sampson, J. J. & Friedman, M. Role of pulmonary lymphatics in chronic pulmonary edema. *Circ. Res.* **11**, 966–970 (1962).

173. Lauweryns, J. & Baert, J. Alveolar clearance and the role of the pulmonary lymphatics. *Am. Rev. Respir. Dis.* **115**, 625–683 (1977).

174. Cai, B. *et al.* Effect of supplementing a high-fat, low-carbohydrate enteral formula in COPD patients. *Nutrition* **19**, 229–232 (2003).

175. Sabapathy, S., Morris, N. R. & Schneider, D. A. Ventilatory and gas-exchange responses to incremental exercise performed with reduced muscle glycogen content. *J. Sci. Med. Sport* **9**, 267–273 (2006).

176. Alessandro, R. *et al.* Effects of twenty days of the ketogenic diet on metabolic and respiratory parameters in healthy subjects. *Lung* **193**, 939–945 (2015).

177. Goldberg, E. L. *et al.* Ketogenic diet activates protective γδ T cell responses against influenza virus infection. *Sci. Immunol.* **4**, (2019).

178. Al-Saady, N. M., Blackmore, C. M. & Bennett, D. Nutritional support in patients with acute respiratory failure undergoing artificial ventilation. in *Update 1989* (ed. Vincent, J. L.) 262–269 (Springer, 1989). doi:10.1007/978-3-642-83737-1_32.

179. Masino, S. A. & Rho, J. M. Mechanisms of Ketogenic Diet Action. in *Jasper's Basic Mechanisms of the Epilepsies* (eds. Noebels, J., Avoli, M., Rogawski, M., Olsen, R. W. & Delgado-Escueta, A.) (National Center for Biotechnology Information (US), 2012).

180. Cava, A. L. & Matarese, G. The weight of leptin in immunity. *Nat. Rev. Immunol.* **4**, 371–379 (2004).

181. Malli, F., Papaioannou, A. I., Gourgoulianis, K. I. & Daniil, Z. The role of leptin in the respiratory system: An overview. *Respir. Res.* **11**, 152 (2010).

182. Raper, D., Louveau, A. & Kipnis, J. How do meningeal lymphatic vessels drain the CNS? *Trends Neurosci.* **39**, 581–586 (2016).

183. He, W. *et al.* The anatomy and metabolome of the lymphatic system in the brain in health and disease. *Brain Pathol.* **30**, 392–404 (2020).

184. Iliff, J. J., Goldman, S. A. & Nedergaard, M. Implications of the discovery of brain lymphatic pathways. *Lancet Neurol.* **14**, 977–979 (2015).

185. Aspelund, A. *et al.* A dural lymphatic vascular system that drains brain interstitial fluid and macromolecules. *J. Exp. Med.* **212**, 991–999 (2015).

186. Zhang, J. & Liu, Q. Cholesterol metabolism and homeostasis in the brain. *Protein Cell* **6**, 254–264 (2015).

187. Linetti, A. *et al.* Cholesterol reduction impairs exocytosis of synaptic vesicles. *J. Cell Sci.* **123**, 595–605 (2010).

188. Jessen, N. A., Munk, A. S. F., Lundgaard, I. & Nedergaard, M. The glymphatic system: a beginner's guide. *Neurochem. Res.* **40**, 2583–2599 (2015).

189. Xie, L. *et al.* Sleep drives metabolite clearance from the adult brain. *Science* **342**, 373–377 (2013).

190. Da Mesquita, S. *et al.* Functional aspects of meningeal lymphatics in ageing and Alzheimer's disease. *Nature* **560**, 185–191 (2018).

191. Brzecka, A. *et al.* Sleep disorders associated with Alzheimer's disease: A perspective. *Front. Neurosci.* **12**, (2018).

192. de la Monte, S. M. & Wands, J. R. Alzheimer's disease is type 3 diabetes–evidence reviewed. *J. Diabetes Sci. Technol. Online* **2**, 1101–1113 (2008).

193. Hoyer, S. Oxidative energy metabolism in Alzheimer brain. Studies in early-onset and late-onset cases. *Mol. Chem. Neuropathol.* **16**, 207–224 (1992).

194. Taylor, M. K., Sullivan, D. K., Mahnken, J. D., Burns, J. M. & Swerdlow, R. H. Feasibility and efficacy data from a ketogenic diet intervention in Alzheimer's disease. *Alzheimers Dement. Transl. Res. Clin. Interv.* **4**, 28–36 (2017).

195. Reger, M. A. *et al.* Effects of beta-hydroxybutyrate on cognition in memory-impaired adults. *Neurobiol. Aging* **25**, 311–314 (2004).

196. Henderson, S. T. *et al.* Study of the ketogenic agent AC-1202 in mild to moderate Alzheimer's disease: A randomized, double-blind, placebo-controlled, multicenter trial. *Nutr. Metab.* **6**, 31 (2009).

197. Ota, M. *et al.* Effects of a medium-chain triglyceride-based ketogenic formula on cognitive function in patients with mild-to-moderate Alzheimer's disease. *Neurosci. Lett.* **690**, 232–236 (2019).

198. Krikorian, R. *et al.* Dietary ketosis enhances memory in mild cognitive impairment. *Neurobiol. Aging* **33**, 425.e19-425.e27 (2012).

199. Proserpio, P., Arnaldi, D., Nobili, F. & Nobili, L. Integrating sleep and Alzheimer's disease pathophysiology: Hints for sleep disorders management. *J. Alzheimers Dis.* **63**, 871–886 (2018).

200. Lee, H. *et al.* The effect of body posture on brain glymphatic transport. *J. Neurosci.* **35**, 11034–11044 (2015).

201. Ruipérez, V., Darios, F. & Davletov, B. Alpha-synuclein, lipids and Parkinson's disease. *Prog. Lipid Res.* **49**, 420–428 (2010).

202. Husmann, M., Roedel, C., Leu, A., Koppensteiner, R. & Franzeck, U. Lymphoedema, lymphatic micro-angiopathy and increased lymphatic and interstitial pressure in a patient with Parkinson's disease. *Schweiz. Med. Wochenschr.* **129**, 410–2 (1999).

203. Leibson, C. L. *et al.* Comorbid conditions associated with Parkinson's disease: A population-based study. *Mov. Disord. Off. J. Mov. Disord. Soc.* **21**, 446–455 (2006).

204. Włodarek, D. Role of ketogenic diets in neurodegenerative diseases (Alzheimer's disease and Parkinson's disease). *Nutrients* **11**, 169 (2019).

205. Sharon, R. *et al.* The formation of highly soluble oligomers of α-synuclein is regulated by fatty acids and enhanced in Parkinson's disease. *Neuron* **37**, 583–595 (2003).

206. Phillips, M. C. L., Murtagh, D. K. J., Gilbertson, L. J., Asztely, F. J. S. & Lynch, C. D. P. Low-fat versus ketogenic diet in Parkinson's disease: A pilot randomized controlled trial. *Mov. Disord.* **33**, 1306–1314 (2018).

207. VanItallie, T. B. *et al.* Treatment of Parkinson disease with diet-induced hyperketonemia: A feasibility study. *Neurology* **64**, 728–730 (2005).

208. Alexander, J. S., Ganta, V. C., Jordan, P. A. & Witte, M. H. Gastrointestinal lymphatics in health and disease. *Pathophysiology* **17**, 315–335 (2010).

209. Ge, Y., Li, Y., Gong, J. & Zhu, W. Mesenteric organ lymphatics and inflammatory bowel disease. *Ann. Anat. – Anat. Anz.* **218**, 199–204 (2018).

210. Miller, M. J. & Newberry, R. D. Microanatomy of the intestinal lymphatic system. *Ann. N. Y. Acad. Sci.* **1207**, E21–E28 (2010).

211. Rehal, S., Stephens, M., Roizes, S., Liao, S. & von der Weid, P.-Y. Acute small intestinal inflammation results in persistent lymphatic alterations. *Am. J. Physiol.-Gastrointest. Liver Physiol.* **314**, G408–G417 (2018).

212. Tran, C. D. *et al.* Gut permeability, its interaction with gut microflora and effects on metabolic health are mediated by the lymphatics system, liver and bile acid. *Future Microbiol.* **10**, 1339–1353 (2015).

213. Heatley, R. V., Bolton, P. M., Hughes, L. E. & Owen, E. W. Mesenteric lymphatic obstruction in Crohn's disease. *Digestion* **20**, 307–313 (1980).

214. Kovi, J., Duong, H. D. & Hoang, C. T. Ultrastructure of intestinal lymphatics in Crohn's disease. *Am. J. Clin. Pathol.* **76**, 385–394 (1981).

215. von der Weid, P.-Y., Rehal, S. & Ferraz, J. G. Role of the lymphatic system in the pathogenesis of Crohn's disease: *Curr. Opin. Gastroenterol.* **27**, 335–341 (2011).

216. Kasper, H. & Sommer, H. Dietary fiber and nutrient intake in Crohn's disease. *Am. J. Clin. Nutr.* **32**, 1898–1901 (1979).

217. Cohen, S. A. *et al.* Clinical and mucosal improvement with specific carbohydrate diet in pediatric Crohn's disease. *J. Pediatr. Gastroenterol. Nutr.* **59**, 516–521 (2014).

218. Donnellan, C. F., Yann, L. H. & Lal, S. Nutritional management of Crohn's disease. *Ther. Adv. Gastroenterol.* **6**, 231–242 (2013).

219. Olendzki, B. C. *et al.* An anti-inflammatory diet as treatment for inflammatory bowel disease: A case series report. *Nutr. J.* **13**, 5 (2014).

220. Tóth, C., Dabóczi, A., Howard, M., J. Miller, N. & Clemens, Z. Crohn's disease successfully treated with the paleolithic ketogenic diet. *Int. J. Case Rep. Images* **7**, 570 (2016).

221. Barton, S. H., Kelly, D. G. & Murray, J. A. Nutritional deficiencies in celiac disease. *Gastroenterol. Clin. North Am.* **36**, 93–108 (2007).

222. Di Sabatino, A., Brunetti, L., Carnevale Maffè, G., Giuffrida, P. & Corazza, G. R. Is it worth investigating splenic function in patients with celiac disease? *World J. Gastroenterol. WJG* **19**, 2313–2318 (2013).

223. Matuchansky, C. *et al.* Cavitation of mesenteric lymph nodes, splenic atrophy, and a flat small intestinal mucosa: Report of six cases. *Gastroenterology* **87**, 606–614 (1984).

224. Leinonen, H. *et al.* Daily life restrictions are common and associated with health concerns and dietary challenges in adult celiac disease patients diagnosed in childhood. *Nutrients* **11**, 1718 (2019).

225. Niewinski, M. M. Advances in celiac disease and gluten-free diet. *J. Am. Diet. Assoc.* **108**, 661–672 (2008).

226. Wacklin, P. *et al.* Altered duodenal microbiota composition in celiac disease patients suffering from persistent symptoms on a long-term gluten-free diet. *Off. J. Am. Coll. Gastroenterol. ACG* **109**, 1933–1941 (2014).

227. Thomas, S. N. *et al.* Impaired humoral immunity and tolerance in K14-VEGFR-3-IG mice that lack dermal lymphatic drainage. *J. Immunol.* **189**, 2181–2190 (2012).

228. Mortimer, P. S. & Rockson, S. G. New developments in clinical aspects of lymphatic disease. *J. Clin. Invest.* **124**, 915–921 (2014).

229. Schwartz, N. *et al.* Lymphatic function in autoimmune diseases. *Front. Immunol.* **10**, (2019).

230. Guo, R. *et al.* Inhibition of lymphangiogenesis and lymphatic drainage via vascular endothelial growth factor receptor 3 blockade increases the severity of inflammation in a mouse model of chronic inflammatory arthritis. *Arthritis Rheum.* **60**, 2666–2676 (2009).

231. Khanna, S., Jaiswal, K. S. & Gupta, B. Managing rheumatoid arthritis with dietary interventions. *Front. Nutr.* **4**, 52 (2017).

232. Kjeldsen-Kragh, J. *et al.* Controlled trial of fasting and one-year vegetarian diet in rheumatoid arthritis. *Lancet Lond. Engl.* **338**, 899–902 (1991).

233. Tedeschi, S. K. & Costenbader, K. H. Is there a role for diet in the therapy of rheumatoid arthritis? *Curr. Rheumatol. Rep.* **18**, 23 (2016).

234. Davies, R. *et al.* Weight loss and improvements in fatigue in systemic lupus erythematosus: a controlled trial of a low glycaemic index diet versus a calorie restricted diet in patients treated with corticosteroids. *Lupus* **21**, 649–655 (2012).

235. Arpaia, G. *et al.* Effects of elastic compression on hypomobility edema and fibrinolysis activation in multiple sclerosis. *Panminerva Med.* **53**, 71–74 (2011).

236. Storoni, M. & Plant, G. T. The therapeutic potential of the ketogenic diet in treating progressive multiple sclerosis. *Mult. Scler. Int.* **2015**, e681289 (2015).

237. Furtado, G. C. *et al.* Lymphotoxin beta receptor signaling is required for inflammatory lymphangiogenesis in the thyroid. *PNAS* **104**, 5026–5031 (2007).

238. Serres-Créixams, X. *et al.* Paratracheal lymph nodes: A new sonographic finding in autoimmune thyroiditis. *J. Clin. Ultrasound* **36**, 418–421 (2008).

239. Fothergill, E. *et al.* Persistent metabolic adaptation 6 years after "The Biggest Loser" competition. *Obesity* **24**, 1612–1619 (2016).

240. Najarian, T. & Rowsemitt, C. N. Hypothyroidism, particularly associated with weight loss: evaluation and treatment based on symptoms and thyroid hormone levels. *Thyroid Sci.* **6**, CR1-7 (2011).

241. Kose, E., Guzel, O. & Arslan, N. Analysis of hematological parameters in patients treated with ketogenic diet due to drug-resistant epilepsy. *Neurol. Sci.* **39**, 85–89 (2018).

242. Keast, D. H., Moffatt, C. & Janmohammad, A. Lymphedema impact and prevalence international study: The Canadian data. *Lymphat. Res. Biol.* **17**, 178–186 (2019).

243. Gordon, S. J. *et al.* LIMPRINT in Australia. *Lymphat. Res. Biol.* **17**, 173–177 (2019).

244. Keeley, V. *et al.* LIMPRINT in specialist lymphedema services in United Kingdom, France, Italy, and Turkey. *Lymphat. Res. Biol.* **17**, 141–146 (2019).

245. Angelantonio, E. D. *et al.* Body-mass index and all-cause mortality: Individual-participant-data meta-analysis of 239 prospective studies in four continents. *The Lancet* **388**, 776–786 (2016).

246. Escobedo, N. & Oliver, G. The lymphatic vasculature: Its role in adipose metabolism and obesity. *Cell Metab.* **26**, 598–609 (2017).

247. Escobedo, N. *et al.* Restoration of lymphatic function rescues obesity in Prox1-haplo insufficient mice. *JCI Insight* **1**, (2016).

248. Harvey, N. L. *et al.* Lymphatic vascular defects promoted by Prox1 haploinsufficiency cause adult-onset obesity. *Nat. Genet.* **37**, 1072–1081 (2005).

249. García Nores, G. D. *et al.* Obesity but not high-fat diet impairs lymphatic function. *Int. J. Obes. 2005* **40**, 1582–1590 (2016).

250. Gousopoulos, E. *et al.* High-fat diet in the absence of obesity does not aggravate surgically induced lymphoedema in mice. *Eur. Surg. Res.* **58**, 180–192 (2017).

251. Ludwig, D. S. The ketogenic diet: Evidence for optimism but high-quality research needed. *J. Nutr.* **150**, 1354–1359 (2020).

252. Bikman, B. *Why We Get Sick.* (BenBella Books, Inc, 2020).

253. Keith, L., Rowsemitt, C. & Richards, L. G. Lifestyle modification group for lymphedema and obesity results in significant health outcomes. *Am. J. Lifestyle Med.* 155982761774210 (2017) doi:10.1177/1559827617742108.

254. Hall, K. D. Challenges of human nutrition research. *Science* **367**, 1298–1300 (2020).

255. Kirkpatrick, S. I. *et al.* The provision of assistance does not substantially impact the accuracy of 24-hour dietary recalls completed using the automated self-administered 24-h dietary assessment tool among women with low incomes. *J. Nutr.* **149**, 114–122 (2019).

256. Archer, E., Hand, G. A. & Blair, S. N. Validity of U.S. nutritional surveillance: National health and nutrition examination survey caloric energy intake data, 1971–2010. *PLoS ONE* **8**, (2013).

257. Ioannidis, J. P. A. Implausible results in human nutrition research. *BMJ* **347**, f6698–f6698 (2013).

258. Keys, A. *et al.* The Seven Countries study: 2,289 deaths in 15 years. *Prev. Med.* **13**, 141–154 (1984).

259. Taubes, G. *Good Calories, Bad Calories: Fats, Carbs, and the Controversial Science of Diet and Health.* (Random House, Inc, 2008).

260. The Vegan Society. *The Vegan Society* https://www.vegansociety.com/.

261. Wallace, T. C. *et al.* Choline. *Nutr. Today* **53**, 240–253 (2018).

262. Wu, G. Important roles of dietary taurine, creatine, carnosine, anserine and 4-hydroxyproline in human nutrition and health. *Amino Acids* **52**, 329–360 (2020).

263.   Doerge, R. D. & Sheehan, D. Scientists protest soy approval. 4 (1999).

264.   Gedgaudas, N. *Primal Body, Primal Mind: Beyond Paleo for Total Health and a Longer Life*. (Healing Arts Press, 2011).

265.   Cholewski, M., Tomczykowa, M. & Tomczyk, M. A comprehensive review of chemistry, sources and bioavailability of omega-3 fatty acids. *Nutrients* **10**, (2018).

266.   Barthels, F., Meyer, F. & Pietrowsky, R. Orthorexic and restrained eating behaviour in vegans, vegetarians, and individuals on a diet. *Eat. Weight Disord. EWD* **23**, 159–166 (2018).

267.   Dagnelie, P. C. [Nutrition and health—potential health benefits and risks of vegetarianism and limited consumption of meat in the Netherlands]. *Ned. Tijdschr. Geneeskd.* **147**, 1308–1313 (2003).

268.   Hibbeln, J. R., Northstone, K., Evans, J. & Golding, J. Vegetarian diets and depressive symptoms among men. *J. Affect. Disord.* **225**, 13–17 (2018).

269.   Shams-White, M. M. *et al.* Dietary protein and bone health: A systematic review and meta-analysis from the National Osteoporosis Foundation. *Am. J. Clin. Nutr.* **105**, 1528–1543 (2017).

270.   Kopp, W. How western diet and lifestyle drive the pandemic of obesity and civilization diseases. *Diabetes Metab. Syndr. Obes. Targets Ther.* **12**, 2221–2236 (2019).

271.   Moreno-Fernández, S. *et al.* High fat/high glucose diet induces metabolic syndrome in an experimental rat model. *Nutrients* **10**, 1502 (2018).

272.   Davis, C., Bryan, J., Hodgson, J. & Murphy, K. Definition of the Mediterranean diet: A literature review. *Nutrients* **7**, 9139–9153 (2015).

273.   Estruch, R. *et al.* Primary prevention of cardiovascular disease with a Mediterranean diet supplemented with extra-virgin olive oil or nuts. *N. Engl. J. Med.* **378**, e34 (2018).

274.   Shively, C. A. *et al.* Mediterranean versus Western diet effects on caloric intake, obesity, metabolism, and hepatosteatosis in nonhuman primates. *Obes.* Silver Spring MD **27**, 777–784 (2019).

275.   Paoli, A., Cenci, L. & Grimaldi, K. A. Effect of ketogenic Mediterranean diet with phytoextracts and low carbohydrates/high-protein meals on weight, cardiovascular risk factors, body composition and diet compliance in Italian council employees. *Nutr. J.* **10**, 112 (2011).

276.   Volek, J. S. & Sharman, M. J. Cardiovascular and hormonal aspects of very-low-carbohydrate ketogenic diets. *Obes. Res.* **12 Suppl 2**, 115S–23S (2004).

277.   Johnson. The paleo diet and the American weight loss utopia, 1975–2014. *Utop. Stud.* **26**, 101 (2015).

278.   Eaton, S. B. & Konner, M. Paleolithic nutrition: A consideration of Its nature and current implications. *N. Engl. J. Med.* **312**, 283–289 (1985).

279.   Kuhn, S. The culture of Crossfit: A lifestyle prescription for optimal health and fitness. *Sr. Theses – Anthropol. Ill. State Univ.* **1**, 15 (2013).

280.   Schwitzer, C., Polowinsky, S. Y. & Solman, C. Fruits as foods – Common misconceptions about frugivory. *5th Eur. Zoo Nutr. Conf.* (2008).

281. Dashti, H. M. *et al.* Long-term effects of a ketogenic diet in obese patients. *Exp. Clin. Cardiol.* **9**, 200–205 (2004).

282. Dressler, A. *et al.* Type 1 diabetes and epilepsy: Efficacy and safety of the ketogenic diet. *Epilepsia* **51**, 1086–1089 (2010).

283. Banting, W. *Letter on corpulence.* (Harrison, 59, Pall Mall, 1864).

284. Cordain, L. *et al.* Origins and evolution of the Western diet: Health implications for the 21st century. *Am. J. Clin. Nutr.* **81**, 341–354 (2005).

285. O'Hearn, A. *Eat Meat. Not Too Little. Mostly Fat. - The Facultative Carnivore.* (2018).

286. McClellan, W. & DuBois, E. Prolonged meat diets with a study of kidney function and ketosis. *J. Biol. Chem.* **87**, 651–668 (1930).

287. Krause, M. R. & Regen, S. L. The structural role of cholesterol in cell membranes: From condensed bilayers to lipid rafts. *Acc. Chem. Res.* **47**, 3512–3521 (2014).

288. Ortolani, C. & Pastorello, E. A. Food allergies and food intolerances. *Best Pract. Res. Clin. Gastroenterol.* **20**, 467–483 (2006).

289. Hallberg, L. Bioavailable nutrient density: A new concept applied in the interpretation of food iron absorption data. *Am. J. Clin. Nutr.* **34**, 2242–2247 (1981).

290. Pawlak, R., Parrott, S. J., Raj, S., Cullum-Dugan, D. & Lucus, D. How prevalent is vitamin B_{12} deficiency among vegetarians? *Nutr. Rev.* **71**, 110–117 (2013).

291. Smith, A. M. Veganism and osteoporosis: A review of the current literature. *Int. J. Nurs. Pract.* **12**, 302–306 (2006).

292. Benton, D. & Donohoe, R. The influence of creatine supplementation on the cognitive functioning of vegetarians and omnivores. *Br. J. Nutr.* **105**, 1100–1105 (2011).

293. Everaert, I. *et al.* Vegetarianism, female gender and increasing age, but not CNDP1 genotype, are associated with reduced muscle carnosine levels in humans. *Amino Acids* **40**, 1221–1229 (2011).

294. Laidlaw, S. A., Shultz, T. D., Cecchino, J. T. & Kopple, J. D. Plasma and urine taurine levels in vegans. *Am. J. Clin. Nutr.* **47**, 660–663 (1988).

295. Doughman, S. D., Krupanidhi, S. & Sanjeevi, C. B. Omega-3 fatty acids for nutrition and medicine: Considering microalgae oil as a vegetarian source of EPA and DHA. *Curr. Diabetes Rev.* **3**, 198–203 (2007).

296. Davis, B. C. & Kris-Etherton, P. M. Achieving optimal essential fatty acid status in vegetarians: Current knowledge and practical implications. *Am. J. Clin. Nutr.* **78**, 640S-646S (2003).

297. Gerster, H. Can adults adequately convert alpha-linolenic acid (18:3n-3) to eicosapentaenoic acid (20:5n-3) and docosahexaenoic acid (22:6n-3)? *Int. J. Vitam. Nutr. Res. Int. Z. Vitam. - Ernahrungsforschung J. Int. Vitaminol. Nutr.* **68**, 159–173 (1998).

298. Hampl, J. S. & Betts, N. M. Comparisons of dietary intake and sources of fat in low – and high-fat diets of 18- to 24-year-olds. *J. Am. Diet. Assoc.* **95**, 893–897 (1995).

299. Lichtenstein, A. H. & Van Horn, L. Very low fat diets. *Circulation* **98**, 935–939 (1998).

300. Ames, B. N., Profet, M. & Gold, L. S. Dietary pesticides (99.99% all natural). *Proc. Natl. Acad. Sci.* **87**, 7777–7781 (1990).

301. Sekhar, J. C. *et al.* Plant toxins-useful and harmful effects. *Hygeia – J. Drugs Med.* **4**, 79–90 (2012).

302. Güzel, A. & Açıkgöz, M. A lethal danger in the home: Turpentine poisoning. *Turk. J. Pediatr.* **57**, 177–179 (2015).

303. Astley, S. & Finglas, P. Nutrition and Health. In *Reference Module in Food Science* B9780081005965033000 (Elsevier, 2016). doi:10.1016/B978-0-08-100596-5.03425-9.

304. Menon, V. *et al.* Effect of a very low-protein diet on outcomes: Long-term follow-up of the modification of diet in renal disease (MDRD) study. *Am. J. Kidney Dis.* **53**, 208–217 (2009).

305. Cuenca-Sánchez, M., Navas-Carrillo, D. & Orenes-Piñero, E. Controversies surrounding high-protein diet intake: Satiating effect and kidney and bone health. *Adv. Nutr.* **6**, 260–266 (2015).

306. Weigle, D. S. *et al.* A high-protein diet induces sustained reductions in appetite, ad libitum caloric intake, and body weight despite compensatory changes in diurnal plasma leptin and ghrelin concentrations. *Am. J. Clin. Nutr.* **82**, 41–48 (2005).

307. Wycherley, T. P., Moran, L. J., Clifton, P. M., Noakes, M. Brinkworth, G. D. Effects of energy-restricted high-protein, low-fat compared with standard-protein, low-fat diets: a meta-analysis of randomized controlled trials. *Am. J. Clin. Nutr.* **96**, 1281–1298 (2012).

308. Wolfe, R. R. Protein Summit: Consensus areas and future research. *Am. J. Clin. Nutr.* **87**, 1582S-1583S (2008).

309. Clark, A., Imran, J., Madni, T. & Wolf, S. E. Nutrition and metabolism in burn patients. *Burns Trauma* **5**, 11 (2017).

310. Phinney, S., Bailey, B. & Volek, J. Inflammation, Nutritional Ketosis, and Keto-Immune Modulation: New Insights Into How Virta Can Reverse Type 2 Diabetes. *Virta Health* https://www.virtahealth.com/blog/inflammation-ketosis-diabetes (2020).

311. Kuratko, C. N., Barrett, E. C., Nelson, E. B. & Norman, S. The relationship of docosahexaenoic acid (DHA) with learning and behavior in healthy children: A review. *Nutrients* **5**, 2777–2810 (2013).

312. Kang, J. X. & Weylandt, K. H. Modulation of inflammatory cytokines by omega-3 fatty acids. *Subcell. Biochem.* **49**, 133–143 (2008).

313. Simopoulos, A. P. The importance of the ratio of omega-6/omega-3 essential fatty acids. *Biomed. Pharmacother.* **56**, 365–379 (2002).

314. Cywes, R. Is Lipedema Different from Other Forms of Obesity? (2020). Ketogenic Solution for Lymphatic/Fat Disorders Virtual Symposium

315. Izadi, V., Saraf-Bank, S. & Azadbakht, L. Dietary intakes and leptin concentrations. *ARYA Atheroscler.* **10**, 266–272 (2014).

316. Nespovitaya, N. *et al.* Dynamic assembly and disassembly of functional β-endorphin amyloid fibrils. *J. Am. Chem. Soc.* **138**, 846–856 (2016).

317. Heller, R. F. & Heller, R. F. Hyperinsulinemic obesity and carbohydrate addiction: The missing link is the carbohydrate frequency factor. *Med. Hypotheses* **42**, 307–312 (1994).

318. Avena, N. M., Rada, P. & Hoebel, B. G. Evidence for sugar addiction: Behavioral and neurochemical effects of intermittent, excessive sugar intake. *Neurosci. Biobehav. Rev.* **32**, 20–39 (2008).

319. Chittenden, R. *Physiological Economy in Nutrition with Special Reference to the Minimal Proteid Requirement of the Healthy Man: An Experimental Study.* (Frederick A. Stokes Company, 1904).

320. Weigley, E. S. Average? Ideal? Desirable? A brief overview of height-weight tables in the United States. *J. Am. Diet. Assoc.* **84**, 417–423 (1984).

321. Naiman, T. & Shewfelt, W. *The P:E Diet: Leverage Your Biology to Achieve Optimal Health.* (self-published, 2019).

322. Calder, P. C. Polyunsaturated fatty acids and inflammation. *Biochem. Soc. Trans.* **33**, 423–427 (2005).

323. Ravnskov, U. The questionable role of saturated and polyunsaturated fatty acids in cardiovascular disease. *J. Clin. Epidemiol.* **51**, 443–460 (1998).

324. Malhotra, A., Redberg, R. F. & Meier, P. Saturated fat does not clog the arteries: Coronary heart disease is a chronic inflammatory condition, the risk of which can be effectively reduced from healthy lifestyle interventions. *Br. J. Sports Med.* **51**, 1111–1112 (2017).

325. Frecka, J. M. & Mattes, R. D. Possible entrainment of ghrelin to habitual meal patterns in humans. *Am. J. Physiol.-Gastrointest. Liver Physiol.* **294**, G699–G707 (2008).

326. Al-Saleh, A. M., Corkey, B., Deeney, J., Tornheim, K. & Bauer, E. Effect of artificial sweeteners on insulin secretion, ROS, and oxygen consumption in pancreatic beta cells. *FASEB J.* **25**, 530.1-530.1 (2011).

327. Wise, P. M., Nattress, L., Flammer, L. J. & Beauchamp, G. K. Reduced dietary intake of simple sugars alters perceived sweet taste intensity but not perceived pleasantness. *Am. J. Clin. Nutr.* **103**, 50–60 (2016).

328. Balcı, A. K. *et al.* General characteristics of patients with electrolyte imbalance admitted to emergency department. *World J. Emerg. Med.* **4**, 113–116 (2013).

329. Ehrlich, C. *Lymphedema and Lipedema Nutrition Guide: Foods, Vitamins, Minerals, and Supplements.* (Lymph Notes, 2015).

330. Sigler, M. H. The mechanism of the natriuresis of fasting. *J. Clin. Invest.* **55**, 377–387 (1975).

331. DiNicolantonio, D. J. *The Salt Fix: Why the Experts Got It All Wrong—and How Eating More Might Save Your Life.* (Harmony Books, 2017).

332. Chetty, R. *et al.* The association between income and life expectancy in the United States, 2001-2014. *JAMA* **315**, 1750 (2016).

333. Stewart, Hayden, and Noel Blisard. *Are lower income households willing and able to budget for fruits and vegetables?* U.S. Department of Agriculture, Economic Research Service, ERR-54, January 2008.

334. French, S. A., Tangney, C. C., Crane, M. M., Wang, Y. & Appelhans, B. M. Nutrition quality of food purchases varies by household income: The SHoPPER study. *BMC Public Health* **19**, 231 (2019).

335. Gundersen, C. & Ziliak, J. P. Food insecurity and health outcomes. *Health Aff. (Millwood)* **34**, 1830–1839 (2015).

336. Walker, R. E., Keane, C. R. & Burke, J. G. Disparities and access to healthy food in the United States: A review of food deserts literature. *Health Place* **16**, 876–884 (2010).

337. Kreitzman, S. N., Coxon, A. Y. & Szaz, K. F. Glycogen storage: Illusions of easy weight loss, excessive weight regain, and distortions in estimates of body composition. *Am. J. Clin. Nutr.* **56**, 292S-293S (1992).

338. Rabast, U., Vornberger, K. H. & Ehl, M. Loss of weight, sodium and water in obese persons consuming a high- or low-carbohydrate diet. *Ann. Nutr. Metab.* **25**, 341–349 (1981).

339. Tiwari, S., Riazi, S. & Ecelbarger, C. A. Insulin's impact on renal sodium transport and blood pressure in health, obesity, and diabetes. *Am. J. Physiol.-Ren. Physiol.* **293**, F974–F984 (2007).

340. Tankeu, A. T., Ndip Agbor, V. & Noubiap, J. J. Calcium supplementation and cardiovascular risk: A rising concern. *J. Clin. Hypertens. Greenwich Conn* **19**, 640–646 (2017).

341. Myneni, V. D. & Mezey, E. Regulation of bone remodeling by vitamin K2. *Oral Dis.* **23**, 1021–1028 (2017).

342. Razzaque, M. S. Magnesium: Are we consuming enough? *Nutrients* **10**, 1863 (2018).

343. DeFilippo, C. *et al.* Impact of diet in shaping gut microbiota revealed by a comparative study in children from Europe and rural Africa. *Proc. Natl. Acad. Sci.* **107**, 14691–14696 (2010).

344. Singh, R. K. *et al.* Influence of diet on the gut microbiome and implications for human health. *J. Transl. Med.* **15**, (2017).

345. Tuteja, A. K. *et al.* Development of functional diarrhea, constipation, irritable bowel syndrome, and dyspepsia during and after traveling outside the usa. *Dig. Dis. Sci.* **53**, 271–276 (2008).

346. Westman, E. C. *A Low Carbohydrate, Ketogenic Diet Manual: No Sugar, No Starch Diet.* (CreateSpace Independent Publishing Platform, 2013).

347. Madura, J. A. & DiBaise, J. K. Quick fix or long-term cure? Pros and cons of bariatric surgery. *F1000 Med. Rep.* **4**, (2012).

348. Herzog, K. *et al.* Metabolic effects of gastric bypass surgery: Is it all about calories? *Diabetes* **69**, 2027–2035 (2020).

349. Brantley, P. J. *et al.* Why patients seek bariatric surgery: Does insurance coverage matter? *Obes. Surg.* **24**, 961–964 (2014).

350. Kolotkin, R. L. & Andersen, J. R. A systematic review of reviews: Exploring the relationship between obesity, weight loss and health-related quality of life. *Clin. Obes.* **7**, 273–289 (2017).

351. Opozda, M., Wittert, G. & Chur-Hansen, A. Patients' reasons for and against undergoing Roux-en-Y gastric bypass, adjustable gastric banding, and vertical sleeve gastrectomy. *Surg. Obes. Relat. Dis.* **13**, 1887–1896 (2017).

352. Cambi, M. P. C. *et al.* Post-bariatric surgery weight regain: Evaluation of nutritional profile of candidate patients for endoscopic argon plasma coagulation. *ABCD Arq. Bras. Cir. Dig. São Paulo* **28**, 40–43 (2015).

353. King, W. C. *et al.* Prevalence of alcohol use disorders before and after bariatric surgery. *JAMA J. Am. Med. Assoc.* **307**, 2516–2525 (2012).

354. Meguid, M. M., Glade, M. J. & Middleton, F. A. Weight regain after Roux-en-Y: A significant 20% complication related to PYY. *Nutrition* **24**, 832–842 (2008).

355. Sjöström, L. *et al.* Effects of bariatric surgery on mortality in Swedish obese subjects. *N Engl J Med* 2007; 357:741-752 (2009) doi:10.1056/NEJMoa066254.

356. Svensson, P.-A. *et al.* Alcohol consumption and alcohol problems after bariatric surgery in the swedish obese subjects study. *Obesity* **21**, 2444–2451 (2013).

357. DeLuca. Bariatric diet – what you can (& can't) eat. *Bariatric Surgery Source* https://www.bariatric-surgery-source.com/bariatric-diet.html (2021).

358. Forbes, R. *et al.* Essential fatty acid plasma profiles following gastric bypass and adjusted gastric banding bariatric surgeries. *Obes. Surg.* **26**, 1237–1246 (2016).

359. Sethi, M. *et al.* Long-term outcomes after biliopancreatic diversion with and without duodenal switch: 2-, 5-, and 10-year data. *Surg. Obes. Relat. Dis. Off. J. Am. Soc. Bariatr. Surg.* **12**, 1697–1705 (2016).

360. Busetto, L. *et al.* Practical Recommendations of the Obesity Management Task Force of the European Association for the Study of Obesity for the Post-Bariatric Surgery Medical Management. *Obes. Facts* **10**, 597–632 (2017).

361. Odom, J. *et al.* Behavioral predictors of weight regain after bariatric surgery. *Obes. Surg.* **20**, 349–356 (2010).

362. Lee, J. Y. J., Keane, M. G. & Pereira, S. Diagnosis and treatment of gallstone disease. *The Practitioner* **259**, 15–19, 2 (2015).

363. Bonfrate, L., Wang, D. Q.-H., Garruti, G. & Portincasa, P. Obesity and the risk and prognosis of gallstone disease and pancreatitis. *Best Pract. Res. Clin. Gastroenterol.* **28**, 623–635 (2014).

364. Festi, D. *et al.* Gallbladder motility and gallstone formation in obese patients following very low calorie diets. Use it (fat) to lose it (well). *Int. J. Obes. Relat. Metab. Disord. J. Int. Assoc. Study Obes.* **22**, 592–600 (1998).

365. Gebhard, R. L. *et al.* The role of gallbladder emptying in gallstone formation during diet-induced rapid weight loss. *Hepatology* **24**, 544–548 (1996).

366. Fobi, M. *et al.* Prophylactic cholecystectomy with gastric bypass operation: Incidence of gallbladder disease. *Obes. Surg.* **12**, 350–353 (2002).

367. Stokes, C. S., Gluud, L. L., Casper, M. & Lammert, F. Ursodeoxycholic acid and diets higher in fat prevent gallbladder stones during weight loss: A meta-analysis of randomized controlled trials. *Clin. Gastroenterol. Hepatol. Off. Clin. Pract. J. Am. Gastroenterol. Assoc.* **12**, 1090-1100.e2; quiz e61 (2014).

368. Davis, E. Gall Bladder Diet: is Keto a Good Choice? *Ketogenic Diet Resource* https://www.ketogenic-diet-resource.com/gall-bladder-diet.html (2020).

369. Bulmer, E. The menace of obesity. *Br. Med. J.* **1**, 1024–1026 (1932).

370. Kemp, R. Carbohydrate addiction. *Practitioner* **190**, 358–364 (1963).

371. Ben-Dor, M., Gopher, A., Hershkovitz, I. & Barkai, R. Man the fat hunter: The demise of homo erectus and the emergence of a new hominin lineage in the middle Pleistocene (ca. 400 kyr) Levant. *PLOS ONE* **6**, e28689 (2011).

372. Anton, S. D. *et al.* Flipping the metabolic switch: Understanding and applying the health benefits of fasting. *Obesity* **26**, 254–268 (2018).

373. Bergqvist, A. G. C., Schall, J. I., Gallagher, P. R., Cnaan, A. & Stallings, V. A. Fasting versus gradual initiation of the ketogenic diet: A prospective, randomized clinical trial of efficacy. *Epilepsia* **46**, 1810–1819 (2005).

374. Finnell, J. S., Saul, B. C., Goldhamer, A. C. & Myers, T. R. Is fasting safe? A chart review of adverse events during medically supervised, water-only fasting. *BMC Complement. Altern. Med.* **18**, (2018).

375. Benoit, F. L. Changes in body composition during weight reduction in obesity: Balance studies comparing effects of fasting and a ketogenic diet. *Ann. Intern. Med.* **63**, 604 (1965).

376. Mehanna, H. M., Moledina, J. & Travis, J. Refeeding syndrome: What it is, and how to prevent and treat it. *BMJ* **336**, 1495–1498 (2008).

377. Yoo, J. H. No clear winner: Effects of the biggest loser on the stigmatization of obese persons. *Health Commun.* **28**, 294–303 (2013).

378. Eckel, R. H. & Yost, T. J. Weight reduction increases adipose tissue lipoprotein lipase responsiveness in obese women. *J. Clin. Invest.* **80**, 992–997 (1987).

379. Durrer, C. *et al.* Short-term low-carbohydrate high-fat diet in healthy young males renders the endothelium susceptible to hyperglycemia-induced damage, an exploratory analysis. *Nutrients* **11**, (2019).

380. Forsythe, C. E. *et al.* Limited effect of dietary saturated fat on plasma saturated fat in the context of a low carbohydrate diet. *Lipids* **45**, 947–962 (2010).

381. Youm, Y.-H. *et al.* The ketone metabolite β-hydroxybutyrate blocks NLRP3 inflammasome-mediated inflammatory disease. *Nat. Med.* **21**, 263–269 (2015).

382. Keith, L. *et al.* Ketogenic diet as a potential intervention for lipedema. *Med. Hypotheses* **146**, 110435 (2021).

383. Finkler, E., Heymsfield, S. B. & St-Onge, M.-P. Rate of weight loss can be predicted by patient characteristics and intervention strategies. *J. Acad. Nutr. Diet.* **112**, 75–80 (2012).

384. Fettke, B. History of Corporate Interest in the Dietary Guidelines. (2020). Ketogenic Solution for Lymphatic/Fat Disorders Virtual Symposium

385. Banta, J. E. *et al.* The global influence of the Seventh-Day Adventist church on diet. *Religions* **9**, 251 (2018).

386. Brown, A. W., Ioannidis, J. P. A., Cope, M. B., Bier, D. M. & Allison, D. B. Unscientific beliefs about scientific topics in nutrition. *Adv. Nutr.* **5**, 563–565 (2014).

387. Nickerson, R. S. Confirmation bias: A ubiquitous phenomenon in many guises. *Rev. Gen. Psychol.* **2**, 175–220 (1998).

388. Astrup, A. A changing view on saturated fatty acids and dairy: From enemy to friend. *Am. J. Clin. Nutr.* **100**, 1407–1408 (2014).

389. Ramsden, C. E. *et al.* Re-evaluation of the traditional diet-heart hypothesis: Analysis of recovered data from Minnesota Coronary Experiment (1968-73). *BMJ* **353**, i1246 (2016).

390. Olsson, A. G. *et al.* Can LDL cholesterol be too low? Possible risks of extremely low levels. *J. Intern. Med.* **281**, 534–553 (2017).

391. Sachdeva, A. *et al.* Lipid levels in patients hospitalized with coronary artery disease: An analysis of 136,905 hospitalizations in Get With The Guidelines. *Am. Heart J.* **157**, 111-117.e2 (2009).

392. Stefansson, V. *The Fat of the Land.* (The MacMillan Company, 1960).

393. Zinn, C., Wood, M., Williden, M., Chatterton, S. & Maunder, E. Ketogenic diet benefits body composition and well-being but not performance in a pilot case study of New Zealand endurance athletes. *J. Int. Soc. Sports Nutr.* **14**, (2017).

394. Harvey, C., Schofield, G. & Willeden, M. The lived experience of healthy adults following a ketogenic diet: A qualitative study. *J. Holist. Perform.* (2018).

395. Khodabakhshi, A., Seyfried, T. N., Kalamian, M., Beheshti, M. & Davoodi, S. H. Does a ketogenic diet have beneficial effects on quality of life, physical activity or biomarkers in patients with breast cancer: A randomized controlled clinical trial. *Nutr. J.* **19**, 87 (2020).

396. McClernon, F. J., Yancy, W. S., Eberstein, J. A., Atkins, R. C. & Westman, E. C. The effects of a low-carbohydrate ketogenic diet and a low-fat diet on mood, hunger, and other self-reported symptoms. *Obesity* **15**, 182–182 (2007).

397. Schmidt, M., Pfetzer, N., Schwab, M., Strauss, I. & Kämmerer, U. Effects of a ketogenic diet on the quality of life in 16 patients with advanced cancer: A pilot trial. *Nutr. Metab.* **8**, 54 (2011).

398. Heaney, R. P. & Layman, D. K. Amount and type of protein influences bone health. *Am. J. Clin. Nutr.* **87**, 1567S-1570S (2008).

399. Kesl, S. *et al.* Sustaining dietary ketosis to improve blood flow and wound healing in young and aged Fisher rats (734.7). *FASEB J.* **28**, 734.7 (2014).

400. Boris, M., Weindorf, S., Lasinski, B. & Boris, G. Lymphedema reduction by noninvasive complex lymphedema therapy. *Oncol. Williston Park N* **8**, 95–106; discussion 109-110 (1994).

401. Kwan, M. L., Cohn, J. C., Armer, J. M., Stewart, B. R. & Cormier, J. N. Exercise in patients with lymphedema: A systematic review of the contemporary literature. *J. Cancer Surviv.* **5**, 320–336 (2011).

402. Schmitz, K. H. Balancing lymphedema risk: Exercise versus deconditioning for breast cancer survivors. *Exerc. Sport Sci. Rev.* **38**, 17–24 (2010).

403. Schmitz, K. H. *et al.* Physical activity and lymphedema (the PAL trial): Assessing the safety of progressive strength training in breast cancer survivors. *Contemp. Clin. Trials* **30**, 233–245 (2009).

404. Winters-Stone, K. M., Laudermilk, M., Woo, K., Brown, J. C. & Schmitz, K. H. Influence of weight training on skeletal health of breast cancer survivors with or at risk for breast cancer-related lymphedema. *J. Cancer Surviv.* **8**, 260–268 (2014).

405. Baumann, F. T., Reike, A., Hallek, M., Wiskemann, J. & Reimer, V. Does exercise have a preventive effect on secondary lymphedema in breast cancer patients following local treatment – a systematic review. *Breast Care* **13**, 380–385 (2018).

406. Stick, C., Grau, H. & Witzleb, E. On the edema-preventing effect of the calf muscle pump. *Eur. J. Appl. Physiol.* **59**, 39–47 (1989).

407. Schmid-Schonbein, G. W. Microlymphatics and lymph flow. *Physiol. Rev.* **70**, 987–1028 (1990).

408. Partsch, H. Intermittent pneumatic compression in immobile patients. *Int. Wound J.* **5**, 389–397 (2008).

409. Masino, S. A. & Ruskin, D. N. Ketogenic diets and pain. *J. Child Neurol.* **28**, 993–1001 (2013).

410. Sørlie, V. Lipodiet: Effect of a low-carbohydrate high fat-diet on pain and quality of life in patients with lipedema. (University of Oslo, 2019).

411. Burger, R. *et al.* Wirkung von aqua-cycling als bewegungstherapie bei der diagnose lipödem. *Phlebologie* **48**, 182–186 (2019).

412. Warburton, D. E. R. & Bredin, S. S. D. Health benefits of physical activity: A systematic review of current systematic reviews. *Curr. Opin. Cardiol.* **32**, 541–556 (2017).

413. Gianesini, S. *et al.* A specifically designed aquatic exercise protocol to reduce chronic lower limb edema. *Phlebol. J. Venous Dis.* **32**, 594–600 (2017).

414. Tidhar, D., Drouin, J. & Shimony, A. Aqua lymphatic therapy in managing lower extremity lymphedema. *J. Support. Oncol.* **5**, 5 (2007).

415. Becker, B. E. Aquatic therapy: Scientific foundations and clinical rehabilitation applications. *PM&R* **1**, 859–872 (2009).

416. Wilcock, I. M., Cronin, J. B. & Hing, W. A. Physiological response to water immersion: A method for sport recovery? *Sports Med.* **36**, 747–765 (2006).

417. Birkenfeld, A. L. *et al.* Lipid mobilization with physiological atrial natriuretic peptide concentrations in humans. *J. Clin. Endocrinol. Metab.* **90**, 3622–3628 (2005).

418. Nestor, J. *Breath: The New Science of a Lost Art.* (Riverhead Books, 2020).

419. Pillar, N. Does breathing have an influence on lymphatic drainage? **1**, 86–88 (2006).

420. Douglass, J., Graves, P. & Gordon, S. Self-care for management of secondary lymphedema: A systematic review. *PLoS Negl. Trop. Dis.* **10**, (2016).

421. Bordoni, B. & Zanier, E. Anatomic connections of the diaphragm: Influence of respiration on the body system. *J. Multidiscip. Healthc.* **6**, 281–291 (2013).

422. Cai, Y., Goldberg, A. N. & Chang, J. L. The nose and nasal breathing in sleep apnea. *Otolaryngol. Clin. North Am.* **53**, 385–395 (2020).

423. Bohlen, H. G., Gasheva, O. Yu. & Zawieja, D. C. Nitric oxide formation by lymphatic bulb and valves is a major regulatory component of lymphatic pumping. *Am. J. Physiol.-Heart Circ. Physiol.* **301**, H1897–H1906 (2011).

424. Dickstein, J., Hay, J., Lue, F. & Moldofsky, H. The relationship of lymphocytes in blood and in lymph to sleep/wake states in sheep. *Sleep* **23**, 185–90 (2000).

425. Zerbe, R., Stropes, L. & Robertson, G. Vasopressin function in the syndrome of inappropriate antidiuresis. *Annu. Rev. Med.* **31**, 315–327 (1980).

426. Iacovides, S., Goble, D., Paterson, B. & Meiring, R. M. Three consecutive weeks of nutritional ketosis has no effect on cognitive function, sleep, and mood compared with a high-carbohydrate, low-fat diet in healthy individuals: A randomized, crossover, controlled trial. *Am. J. Clin. Nutr.* **110**, 349–357 (2019).

427. Afaghi, A., O'Connor, H. & Chow, C. M. Acute effects of the very low carbohydrate diet on sleep indices. *Nutr. Neurosci.* **11**, 146–154 (2008).

428. Castro, A. I. *et al.* Effect of a very low-calorie ketogenic diet on food and alcohol cravings, physical and sexual activity, sleep disturbances, and quality of life in obese patients. *Nutrients* **10**, 1348 (2018).

429. Hallböök, T., Lundgren, J. & Rosén, I. Ketogenic diet improves sleep quality in children with therapy-resistant epilepsy. *Epilepsia* **48**, 59–65 (2007).

430. Willi, S. M., Oexmann, M. J., Wright, N. M., Collop, N. A. & Key, L. L. The effects of a high-protein, low-fat, ketogenic diet on adolescents with morbid obesity: Body composition, blood chemistries, and sleep abnormalities. *Pediatrics* **101**, 61–67 (1998).

431. Husain, A. M., Yancy, W. S., Carwile, S. T., Miller, P. P. & Westman, E. C. Diet therapy for narcolepsy. *Neurology* **62**, 2300–2302 (2004).

432. Jamieson, J. P., Mendes, W. B. & Nock, M. K. Improving acute stress responses: The power of reappraisal. *Curr. Dir. Psychol. Sci.* **22**, 51–56 (2013).

433. Sherman, K. A., Miller, S. M., Roussi, P. & Taylor, A. Factors predicting adherence to risk management behaviors of women at increased risk for developing lymphedema. *Support. Care Cancer* **23**, 61–69 (2015).

434. Shannon, A. D., Quin, J. W. & Jones, M. a. S. Response of the regional lymphatic system of the sheep to acute stress and adrenaline. *Q. J. Exp. Physiol. Cogn. Med. Sci.* **61**, 169–183 (1976).

435. Segerstrom, S. C. & Miller, G. E. Psychological stress and the human immune system: A meta-analytic study of 30 years of inquiry. *Psychol. Bull.* **130**, 601–630 (2004).

436. Le, C. P. *et al.* Chronic stress in mice remodels lymph vasculature to promote tumour cell dissemination. *Nat. Commun.* **7**, 10634 (2016).

437. Honguten, A., Mekhora, K., Pichaiyongwongdee, S. & Somprasong, S. Effects of lymphatic drainage therapy on autonomic nervous system responses in healthy subjects: A single blind randomized controlled trial. *J. Bodyw. Mov. Ther.* **0**, (2021).

438. Bostock, E. C. S., Kirkby, K. C. & Taylor, B. V. M. The current status of the ketogenic diet in psychiatry. *Front. Psychiatry* **8**, (2017).

439.   Brownlow, M. L., Jung, S. H., Moore, R. J., Bechmann, N. & Jankord, R. Nutritional ketosis affects metabolism and behavior in sprague-dawley rats in both control and chronic stress environments. *Front. Mol. Neurosci.* **10**, (2017).

440.   Nair, R. & Maseeh, A. Vitamin D: The "sunshine" vitamin. *J. Pharmacol. Pharmacother.* **3**, 118–126 (2012).

441.   Humble, M. B. Vitamin D, light and mental health. *J. Photochem. Photobiol. B* **101**, 142–149 (2010).

442.   Gunville, C., M. Mourani, P. & A. Ginde, A. The role of vitamin D in prevention and treatment of infection. *Inflamm. Allergy – Drug Targets Former. Curr. Drug Targets – Inflamm. Allergy* **12**, 239–245 (2013).

443.   Lambert, G., Reid, C., Kaye, D., Jennings, G. & Esler, M. Effect of sunlight and season on serotonin turnover in the brain. *The Lancet* **360**, 1840–1842 (2002).

444.   Young, S. N. How to increase serotonin in the human brain without drugs. *J. Psychiatry Neurosci. JPN* **32**, 394–399 (2007).

445.   Nakade, M., Takeuchi, H., Taniwaki, N., Noji, T. & Harada, T. An integrated effect of protein intake at breakfast and morning exposure to sunlight on the circadian typology in Japanese infants aged 2–6 years. *J. Physiol. Anthropol.* **28**, 239–245 (2009).

446.   Dimech, M. A. Melatonin and sleep disorders: The neurobiology of sleep, circadian rhythm sleep disorders, and various treatment methods. *Inq. J.* **5**, (2013).

447.   Reiter, R. J., Tan, D., Osuna, C. & Gitto, E. Actions of melatonin in the reduction of oxidative stress. *J. Biomed. Sci.* **7**, 444–458 (2000).

448.   Xie, S., Fan, W., He, H. & Huang, F. Role of melatonin in the regulation of pain. *J. Pain Res.* **13**, 331–343 (2020).

449.   El-Missiry, M. A., El-Missiry, Z. M. A. & Othman, A. I. Melatonin is a potential adjuvant to improve clinical outcomes in individuals with obesity and diabetes with coexistence of Covid-19. *Eur. J. Pharmacol.* **882**, 173329 (2020).

450.   Pizzo, P. A. A prescription for longevity in the 21st century: Renewing purpose, building and sustaining social engagement, and embracing a positive lifestyle. *JAMA* **323**, 415 (2020).

451.   Martino, J., Pegg, J. & Frates, E. P. The connection prescription: Using the power of social interactions and the deep desire for connectedness to empower health and wellness. *Am. J. Lifestyle Med.* **11**, 466–475 (2017).

452.   Holt-Lunstad, J., Smith, T. B. & Layton, J. B. Social relationships and mortality risk: A meta-analytic review. *PLOS Med.* **7**, e1000316 (2010).

453.   Griffiths, R. *et al.* Assessment of health, well-being and social connections: A survey of women living in Western Sydney. *Int. J. Nurs. Pract.* **13**, 3–13 (2007).

454.   Boehm, J. & Kubzansky, L. The heart's content: The association between positive psychological well-being and cardiovascular health. *Psychol. Bull.* **138**, 655–91 (2012).

455.   Cohen, S., Alper, C. M., Doyle, W. J., Treanor, J. J. & Turner, R. B. Positive emotional style predicts resistance to illness after experimental exposure to rhinovirus or influenza a virus. *Psychosom. Med.* **68**, 809–815 (2006).

456. Steptoe, A., O'Donnell, K., Badrick, E., Kumari, M. & Marmot, M. Neuroendocrine and inflammatory factors associated with positive affect in healthy men and women: The Whitehall II study. *Am. J. Epidemiol.* **167**, 96–102 (2008).

457. Kok, B. E. *et al.* How positive emotions build physical health: Perceived positive social connections account for the upward spiral between positive emotions and vagal tone. *Psychol. Sci.* **24**, 1123–1132 (2013).

458. McMahon, E. The Emotional Challenges of a Fat Disorder. (2017). Fat Disorders Research Society Conference

459. Gardner, B., Lally, P. & Wardle, J. Making health habitual: The psychology of 'habit-formation' and general practice. *Br. J. Gen. Pract.* **62**, 664–666 (2012).

460. Lally, P., van Jaarsveld, C. H. M., Potts, H. W. W. & Wardle, J. How are habits formed: Modelling habit formation in the real world. *Eur. J. Soc. Psychol.* **40**, 998–1009 (2010).

461. Lally, P. & Gardner, B. Promoting habit formation. *Health Psychol. Rev.* **7**, S137–S158 (2013).

462. Mekarski, J.E. Essential hypertension is lymphatic: a working hypothesis. *Med Hypotheses*. 1998 Aug;51(2):101-3.

463. Boonstra, R. Reality as the leading cause of stress: Rethinking the impact of chronic stress in nature. *Functional Ecology*, 27(1), 2013: 11-23. Retrieved July 4, 2021, from http://www.jstor.org/stable/23480529

464. Casley-Smith JR. The phylogeny of the fine structure of blood vessels and lymphatics: similarities and differences. *Lymphology*. 1987 Dec;20(4):182-8.

465. Miller AM. Role of IL-33 in inflammation and disease. *J Inflamm* (Lond). 2011 Aug 26;8(1):22. doi: 10.1186/1476-9255-8-22.

466. Lee Y, Fluckey JD, Chakraborty S, Muthuchamy M. Hyperglycemia- and hyperinsulinemia-induced insulin resistance causes alterations in cellular bioenergetics and activation of inflammatory signaling in lymphatic muscle. FASEB J. 2017 Jul;31(7):2744-2759.

"By George!" cried the inspector. "How did you ever see that?"
"Because I looked for it."
—Sir Arthur Conan Doyle, *The Adventure of the Dancing Men*

About the Author

Leslyn Keith, OTD, CLT-LANA, has a Clinical Doctorate in Occupational Therapy with an emphasis on lymphedema and obesity. She was certified as a Lymphedema Therapist in 2000 and became LANA-certified in 2001. Dr. Keith has started four lymphedema therapy programs in California including two in private practice.

Currently, Dr. Keith serves as the Director of Research and the President of the Board of Directors for the Lipedema Project, a non-profit organization dedicated to raising awareness, providing education, and supporting research to identify treatment and a cure for lipedema. She also currently consults and lectures on lymphedema, lipedema, and obesity nationally and teaches lymphatic therapy as an instructor for Klose Training.

She can be contacted via email at leslynkeithot@gmail.com and more information about Dr. Keith can be found on her website at leslynkeith.com.

Other Books and Courses by Leslyn Keith, OT

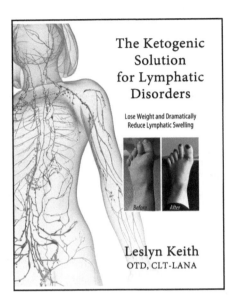

Lymphatic Lifestyle Solutions Course

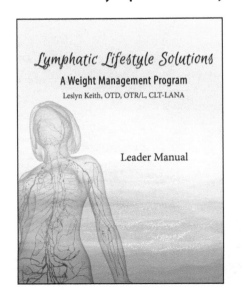

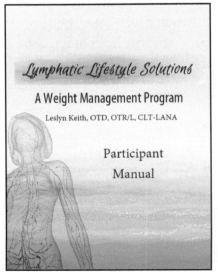